P9-CAJ-953

DEJA REVIEW

USMLE Step 2 Essentials

NOTICE

Medicine is an ever-changing science. As new research and clinical experience broaden our knowledge, changes in treatment and drug therapy are required. The authors and the publisher of this work have checked with sources believed to be reliable in their efforts to provide information that is complete and generally in accord with the standards accepted at the time of publication. However, in view of the possibility of human error or changes in medical sciences, neither the authors nor the publisher nor any other party who has been involved in the preparation or publication of this work warrants that the information contained herein is in every respect accurate or complete, and they disclaim all responsibility for any errors or omissions or for the results obtained from use of the information contained in this work. Readers are encouraged to confirm the information contained herein with other sources. For example and in particular, readers are advised to check the product information sheet included in the package of each drug they plan to administer to be certain that the information contained in this work is accurate and that changes have not been made in the recommended dose or in the contraindications for administration. This recommendation is of particular importance in connection with new or infrequently used drugs.

DEJA REVIEW

USMLE Step 2 Essentials

John H. Naheedy, MD
Resident Radiologist
Department of Radiology
University of California, San Diego
San Diego, California
Class of 2004
College of Medicine
The Ohio State University
Columbus, Ohio

Daniel A. Orringer, MD
Resident Surgeon
Department of Neurosurgery
University of Michigan Medical School
Ann Arbor, Michigan
Class of 2004
College of Medicine
The Ohio State University
Columbus, Ohio

Khashi Mohebali, MD
Resident, Clinical Instructor
Department of Surgery
University of California, San Francisco
San Francisco, California
Class of 2004
College of Medicine
The Ohio State University
Columbus, Ohio

Peter F. Aziz, MD
Resident Physician
Department of Pediatrics
University of Michigan Medical School
Ann Arbor, Michigan
Class of 2004
College of Medicine
The Ohio State University
Columbus, Ohio

Susie Lim, MD
Resident, Clinical Instructor
Department of Obstetrics and Gynecology
The Ohio State University Medical Center
Class of 2004
College of Medicine
The Ohio State University
Columbus, Ohio

LIFE UNIVERSITY
1269 BARCLAY CIRCLE
MARIETTA, GA 30060
(770) 426-2688

WITHDRAWN
LIFE UNIVERSITY
LIBRARY

McGraw-Hill
MEDICAL PUBLISHING DIVISION

New York   Chicago   San Francisco   Lisbon   London   Madrid   Mexico City
Milan   New Delhi   San Juan   Seoul   Singapore   Sydney   Toronto

The **McGraw·Hill** Companies

Deja Review: USMLE Step 2 Essentials

Copyright © 2006 by The McGraw-Hill Companies, Inc. All rights reserved. Printed in the United States of America. Except as permitted under the United States Copyright Act of 1976, no part of this publication may be reproduced or distributed in any form or by any means, or stored in a data base or retrieval system, without the prior written permission of the publisher.

1 2 3 4 5 6 7 8 9 0   DOC/DOC   0 9 8 7 6 5

ISBN: 0-07-144876-4

This book was set in Palatino by International Typesetting and Composition.

The editor was Catherine A. Johnson.

The production supervisor was Catherine Saggese.

The text was designed by Marsha Cohen/Parallelogram.

Project management was provided by International Typesetting and Composition.

RR Donnelley was printer and binder.

This book is printed on acid-free paper.

Library of Congress Cataloging-in-Publication Data

Deja Review : USMLE Step 2 essentials / John H. Naheedy . . . [et al.].
    p. ; cm.
  Includes index.
  ISBN 0-07-144876-4
  1. Clinical medicine—Examinations, questions, etc. 2. Physicians—Licenses—United States—Examinations—Study guides.
    [DNLM: 1. Clinical Medicine—Examination Questions. 2. Specialties, Medical—Examination Questions. WB 18.2 T443 2005] I. Title: USMLE Step 2 essentials. II. Naheedy, John H.
  RC58.T49 2005
  616'.0076—dc22

2004065631

$19.95

To my family and friends,
for their love and encouragement;
and to my parents,
for being an example of everything I want to be.
—John

To my mother and my family.
—Dan

To my parents,
for dedicating and sacrificing their lives
to make mine better;
to my friends,
for their invaluable loyalty;
and to my mentor Dr. Muscarella,
who took the time to put extra effort into a student,
which has meant more to me than he probably realizes.
—Khashi

To my family,
for teaching me that the love of medicine
can be genetically inherited;
and to the bunker, the sand trap of my closest friends,
thanks for the inspiration.
—Pete

To my parents and brother,
for their undying support;
and to my best friend and husband, Mike,
for the love and laughter.
—Susie

Contents

Preface

Step 2 of the United States Medical Licensing Examination (USMLE) tests the senior medical student's ability to apply the basic principles of clinical medicine. However, before you can apply those principles, you must be able to rapidly recall a core body of essential facts. This is why the *Deja Review* series is the most efficient, well-organized, portable, and above all, high-yield resource to prepare students for the USMLE. As recent graduates who have taken Step 2, we are confident that we have compiled a novel review guide that promotes rapid recall of all of the essential facts necessary for success on this examination. We also realize that a solid foundation in these principles will allow you to make a smooth transition into your residency.

ORGANIZATION

All concepts are presented in a question and answer format that covers the key facts on hundreds of common and uncommon diseases. The material is divided into chapters covering the six major divisions of clinical medicine: internal medicine, surgery, neuroscience, psychiatry, OB/GYN, and pediatrics. We have also included a brief emergency medicine chapter that addresses topics not covered under emergent conditions in each of the other chapters.

This question and answer format has several important advantages:
- It provides a rapid, straightforward way for you to assess your strengths and weaknesses.
- It allows you to efficiently review and commit to memory a large body of information.
- It will prepare you for getting "pimped" by residents and attendings on the wards.
- It offers you a break from tedious, convoluted multiple-choice questions.
- The clinical vignettes will expose you to the prototypic presentation of diseases classically tested on the USMLE Step 2.
- It serves as a quick, last-minute review of high-yield facts.

The compact, condensed design of the book is conducive to studying on the go, especially during any downtime on the wards.

HOW TO USE THIS BOOK

Remember, this text is not intended to replace comprehensive textbooks, course packs, or lectures. It is, however, intended to serve as a supplement to your studies during the third and fourth years of medical school. This text has been sampled by a number of medical students who found it to be an essential part of their preparation for the USMLE shelf examinations, in addition to Step 2 itself. We recommend having the text spiral bound to make it more portable and easier to use. Begin using this book early in your third year by carrying it with you during your clinical clerkships. You may cover up the answers and quiz yourself or even your classmates. For a greater challenge, try covering up the questions!

However you choose to study, we hope you find this resource helpful during your preparation for the USMLE Step 2 and throughout your clinical rotations. Best of luck!

John H. Naheedy, MD
Daniel A. Orringer, MD
Khashi Mohebali, MD
Peter F. Aziz, MD
Susie Lim, MD

Acknowledgments

The authors would like to thank the following individuals for their invaluable contributions to this text and their efforts in making this a useful resource for students:

Deborah A. Bartholomew, MD
Clinical Associate Professor
Department of Obstetrics and Gynecology
The Ohio State University Medical Center
Columbus, Ohio

Kathryn Boyse
Resident, Clinical Instructor
Division of Dermatology
The Ohio State University Medical Center
Columbus, Ohio

Megan L. DeHaan, MD
Resident, Clinical Instructor
Department of Radiation Oncology
Kaiser Permanente Los Angeles
   Medical Center
Los Angeles, California

Michael E. Ezzie, MD
Chief Resident, 2004–2005
Department of Internal Medicine
The Ohio State University Medical Center
Columbus, Ohio

Timothy Frankel, MD
Resident Surgeon
Section of General Surgery
Department of Surgery
University of Michigan Medical School
Ann Arbor, Michigan

Bela Gandhi, MD
Resident, Clinical Instructor
Department of Psychiatry
The Ohio State University Medical Center
Columbus, Ohio

Jim Hanje, MD
Clinical Fellow, Digestive Diseases
Department of Internal Medicine
The Ohio State University Medical Center
Columbus, Ohio

Sheri Hart, MD, PhD
Resident, Clinical Instructor
Department of Neurology
The Ohio State University Medical Center
Columbus, Ohio

Stacey Hindy
Resident, Clinical Instructor
Division of Plastic Surgery
The Ohio State University Medical Center
Columbus, Ohio

Peter Muscarella II, MD
Assistant Professor, Clinical
Department of Surgery
The Ohio State University Medical Center
Columbus, Ohio

Emile El-Shammaa, MD
Assistant Professor, Clinical
Department of Emergency Medicine
Department of Pediatrics
Columbia, Ohio
The Ohio State University Medical Center
Columbus, Ohio

Rosemarie Lin Shim, MD
Chief Resident, 2004–2005
Department of Internal Medicine
The Ohio State University Medical Center
Columbus, Ohio

The authors would like to recognize the faculty and staff at The Ohio State University College of Medicine for their endless commitment to education. Without the wisdom and encouragement of mentors like John M. Stang, MD, this project would not have been possible. We would also like to thank the students who used this text in preparation for their boards and provided feedback essential to optimizing this text. Finally, special thanks to David Forrer and his colleagues at Witherspoon Associates, as well as our acquisitions editor, Catherine Johnson, for her patience and guidance throughout this project.

CHAPTER 1

Internal Medicine

CARDIOLOGY

Hypertension

What percentage of hypertensive patients have essential hypertension (HTN)?

90–95%

Name the cause of secondary (2°) HTN in the following clinical scenarios:

HTN upper extremities; decreased or normal blood pressure (BP) in lower extremities

Coarctation of the aorta

HTN accompanied by proteinuria in a nondiabetic patient

Glomerular disease

HTN in a patient with a history of (h/o) renal and hepatic cysts

Polycystic kidney disease

Sudden worsening of HTN in an elderly male with coronary artery disease (CAD) and peripheral vascular disease (PVD)

Renal artery stenosis

Episodic HTN, weight loss, and diaphoresis

Pheochromocytoma

Elevated systolic HTN without diastolic HTN

Hyperthyroidism

40-year-old (y/o) female with a h/o 20 years of oral contraceptive pills (OCP) use

Drug-induced (OCP) HTN

HTN in a patient with hypokalemic metabolic alkalosis

Conn's syndrome/ hyperaldosteronism

HTN in an overweight patient with buffalo hump, moon facies, hirsutism, and abdominal striae

Cushing's syndrome

What is the difference between hypertensive urgency and hypertensive emergency?

In hypertensive urgency there are no signs of end-organ damage due to HTN. In hypertensive emergency there are signs of organ damage

What is the treatment of hypertensive urgency?

Oral BP medication

What are the three preferred agents for the treatment of hypertensive emergency?

IV nitroprusside, nitroglycerine, and hydralazine

For each condition listed below, select the best antihypertensive agent(s):

No comorbidities

Diuretics or β-blockers

Isolated systolic HTN

Thiazide diuretics

Angina pectoris

β-Blockers, Ca^{2+} channel blockers

Diabetes

Angiotensin converting enzyme inhibitors (ACEi) or angiotensin receptor blocker (ARB), β-blockers

Hyperlipidemia

ACEi, Ca^{2+} channel blockers

Congestive heart failure (CHF)

Diuretics, ACEi

H/o myocardial infarction (MI)

β-blockers, ACEi

Chronic renal failure

Diuretics, Ca^{2+} blockers

Asthma, chronic obstructive pulmonary disease (COPD)

Diuretics, Ca^{2+} blockers

Benign prostatic hyperplasia (BPH)

α_1-selective antagonist

Pheochromocytoma

Phenoxybenzamine, phentolamine

Hypertrophic obstructive cardiomyopathy

β-blockers

Hyperthyroidism

β-blockers

Anxiety

β-blockers

Supraventricular tachycardia (SVT)

β-blockers

Migraine headaches

β-blockers, Ca^{2+} blockers

Moderate bradycardia

β-blockers with intrinsic sympathomimetic activity: pindolol and acebutolol

Osteoporosis

Thiazide diuretics

For each condition listed below, list the antihypertensive agent that should be used with caution:

CHF	Verapamil, α-blockers
Asthma, COPD	β-Blockers
Diabetes	β-Blockers, thiazides
Renal artery stenosis, renal failure	ACE inhibitors

Hypercholesterolemia

What genetic disease should be suspected in a patient with xanthomas, xanthelasmas, and lipemia retinalis?	Familial hypercholesterolemia

State the recommended therapeutic intervention or further workup (W/U) for patients with the following lipid values:

Total cholesterol <200	Retest in 5 years
Total cholesterol >200	Treat based on lipid fractions
Low-density lipoprotein (LDL) >190	Begin lipid-lowering therapy
LDL >160 in a patient with two or more coronary risk factors or	Begin lipid-lowering therapy
LDL >130 in a patient with CAD or diabetes mellitus (DM)	Begin lipid-lowering therapy
LDL >100 in a patient with a previous MI	Begin lipid-lowering therapy
Triglycerides (TGs) >200	Begin TG-lowering therapy

For each of the following drugs, provide: (1) the mechanism of action (MOA), (2) indication(s) (IND), and (3) significant side effects and unique toxicity (TOX) (if any):

Cholestyramine	**MOA:** Bile-acid-binding resin
	IND: Adjuvant therapy for patients with familial hypercholesterolemia
	TOX: Constipation, gastrointestinal (GI) discomfort, may interfere with intestinal absorption of other drugs
Statins	**MOA:** Hydroxymethylglutaryl (HMG) coenzyme A (CoA) reductase inhibitors
	IND: Hypercholesterolemia
	TOX: Hepatotoxicity, rhabdomyolysis

Niacin	**MOA:** Reduces release of very low-density lipoprotein (VLDL) from liver into circulation
	IND: Hypercholesterolemia: to ↑ high-density lipoprotein (HDL) and ↓ LDL
	TOX: Flushing, pruritus (both reversible with aspirin), and hepatotoxicity
Gemfibrozil, clofibrate	**MOA:** Stimulates lipoprotein lipase
	IND: Hypercholesterolemia; to ↓↓ TGs
	TOX: Myositis, hepatotoxicity

Coronary Artery Disease

Which are the six coronary risk factors?	**CAD HDL**
	Cigarettes **A**ge (males >45 and females >55 are at increased risk) and sex (males > females)
	Diabetes mellitus (greatest risk factor)
	HTN
	Death from MI in family history (FH) (males <55 y/o, females <60 y/o)
	↑ **L**DL, low HDL (<35)
What is the common presentation of a patient with symptomatic CAD?	Angina pectoris ± radiation to jaw, left shoulder or arm; exacerbated by exertion, relieved by rest, and nitroglycerin
Which groups of patients commonly do *not* exhibit classic anginal symptoms in the setting of myocardial ischemia?	Elderly, women, and diabetics (due to diabetic neuropathy)
Which type of angina is characterized by chest pain and dyspnea at rest?	Unstable angina
What are the classic ECG findings during an anginal episode?	>1 mm ST segment depression and T-wave inversion
What diagnostic tests are often used to screen for CAD?	Exercise or pharmacologic stress test or imaging
What is the gold standard for the diagnosis of CAD?	Coronary arteriography

Name six lifestyle changes that should be suggested to all patients with HTN.

Weight loss, sodium restriction, physical exercise, smoking and alcohol cessation, and stress reduction

What medications should be given to a patient with acute onset of angina?

Sublingual nitroglycerin

What medications should be given as prophylaxis for angina and MI?

Long-acting nitrates, β-blockers, ASA, statin (and ACEi in patients with h/o MI)

What are the key steps in the medical management of a patient with unstable angina?

Start IV, administer O_2, start heparin, ASA, β-blocker, nitroglycerin, morphine

Describe how nitrates reduce angina.

1. Venodilation causes venous pooling $\rightarrow \uparrow$ preload $\rightarrow \uparrow$ myocardial O_2 consumption
2. Coronary vasodilation $\rightarrow \uparrow O_2$ delivery to the myocardium

What is the most common side effect of nitrates?

Headache

Describe how each of the following drugs reduces angina:

β**-Blockers**

$\downarrow$ Myocardial O_2 use, $\downarrow$ afterload, $\uparrow$ coronary filling during diastole

Nifedipine

Coronary arteriolar vasodilation

Verapamil

Slows cardiac conduction

What is the antianginal drug of choice for prinzmetal angina?

Diltiazem

Which antianginal drug must be used with caution in patients with asthma and COPD?

β-blockers

What intervention is reserved for patients whose angina cannot be controlled medically?

Percutaneous transluminal coronary angioplasty (PTCA)

What are the indications for coronary artery bypass grafting?

Angina refractory to medical therapy, severe left main disease, and triple vessel coronary disease (or double vessel disease in a diabetic)

Myocardial Infarction

What is the common presentation of MI?	Crushing retrosternal chest pressure occurring at rest and radiating to left arm, neck or jaw, diaphoresis, nausea/vomiting, dyspnea, anxiety
What is a common physical examination finding during an MI?	S4 gallop
Which are the six life-threatening causes of chest pain that must be ruled out in all patients?	MI, aortic dissection, pulmonary embolism (PE), pneumothorax (PTX), esophageal rupture, cardiac tamponade
What are the key steps in the initial management of a patient with suspected MI?	Assess vital signs, administer O_2, start IV, place on cardiac monitor and obtain ECG; administer ASA, heparin, nitrates, β-blockers, morphine, clopidogrel
What are the classic ECG abnormalities in an acute MI?	ST elevation and Q waves
Which ECG finding is very sensitive and specific for right ventricular infarction?	ST elevation of 1 mm in right-sided lead V4
Which coronary artery is likely to be occluded in a patient with the following ECG abnormalities?	
Large R and ST segment depression in V1, V2	Right coronary (posterior infarction)
Q waves and ST segment elevation in leads V1–V4	Left anterior descending (anterior infarction)
Q wave in leads I, aVL, V5, V6	Circumflex (lateral infarction)
Q waves and ST elevation in leads II, III, aVF	Right coronary (inferior infarction)
Which serologic markers are typically used to diagnose and follow an MI?	Troponin I and CK-MB
What medication is reserved for patients with MI suffering from angina that is refractory to conventional medical management?	Thrombolytics including tissue plasminogen activator or streptokinase
What intervention is indicated in patients during an MI who fail or cannot tolerate thrombolytic therapy?	PTCA

Which medical therapy should be avoided in a patient with a right ventricular infarction?	Nitroglycerin (initial therapy should involve IV fluids to ↑ preload)
What long-term medications have been shown to improve mortality in patients with MI?	ASA and β-blockers (acutely); ACEi, statins, and clopidogrel (long term)

Arrhythmias

Name the arrhythmia associated with the following clinical features:

PR interval >0.2 s, often due to increased vagal tone	Primary (1°) heart block
PR interval gradually increases to the point at which a QRS complex is dropped (P wave is not conducted)	2° Mobitz type I heart block (Wenkebach)
PR interval >0.2 s with occasional dropping of the QRS complex at a fixed interval (i.e., 2:1 or 3:1)	2° Mobitz type II heart block
Irregularly irregular pulses and QRS complexes	Atrial fibrillation
Type of heart block that commonly arises as a side effect of medication including β-blockers, digoxin, and calcium channel blockers	2° Mobitz type II heart block
Sawtooth appearance of P waves	Atrial flutter
Usually caused by conduction block within the bundle of His	2° Mobitz type II heart block
Complete dissociation between P waves and QRS complexes	3° or complete heart block
Three or more P-wave morphologies	Multifocal atrial tachycardia
Associated with cannon A waves in jugular veins and widened pulse pressure	3° heart block
Irregularly irregular pulses and QRS complexes	Atrial fibrillation
Commonly caused by reentry	Paroxsymal SVT
Associated with COPD	Atrial fibrillation, atrial flutter, multifocal atrial tachycardia
Treatment commonly includes anticoagulation, rate control, and/or cardioversion	Atrial fibrillation

Wide QRS complexes not preceded by a P wave	Premature ventricular contraction (PVC)
Normal QRS morphology with a rate of 150–200 beats/min	Paroxsymal SVT
Pharmocologic treatment includes amiodarone, lidocaine, and procainamide	Ventricular tachycardia
May be treated with carotid massage or Valsalva maneuver	Paroxsymal SVT
Common cause of palpitation caused by ectopic beats arising from multiple Ventricular foci	PVC
Ventricular arrhythmia commonly caused by myocardial ischemia that may lead to hemodynamic instability	Ventricular tachycardia
First-line therapy is defibrillation; second-line therapy is epinephrine or vasopressin	Ventricular fibrillation
Polymorphic wide complex tachycardia associated with prolonged QT interval	Torsade de pointes
Treated identical to ventricular fibrillation if there is no pulse	Ventricular tachycardia
Tachyarrhythmia treated with adenosine, verapamil, cardioversion, or radiofrequency ablation	Paroxsymal SVT
Narrow complex tachycardia in which P waves follow QRS	Junctional tachycardia or Wolff-Parkinson-White
Treatment with pacemaker is necessary	Bifascicular $2°$ Mobitz type II heart block, symptomatic $3°$ heart block and sinus node dysfunction
What is the most common cause of atrial fibrillation?	HTN
What are some other important causes of atrial fibrillation?	Pulmonary disease
	Ischemia of myocardium
	Rheumatic heart disease
	Anemia or atrial myxoma
	Thyrotoxicosis
	Ethanol
	Sepsis

Name three clinical scenarios in which atropine is indicated for treatment of a bradyarrhythmia.

1. Bradycardia causing hemodynamic instability
2. Syncope
3. CHF

Congestive Heart Failure

Name six common symptoms of CHF.

1. Dyspnea; exertional initially but occurs at rest as disease progresses
2. Orthopnea
3. Paroxysmal nocturnal dyspnea
4. Cough and wheezing
5. Weight gain due to peripheral edema
6. Worsening fatigue

Name four common signs of left-sided CHF.

1. S3 gallop
2. Inspiratory crackles or rales
3. Laterally displaced point of maximal impulse (due to cardiomegaly)
4. Ventricular heave

Name five common signs of right-sided CHF.

1. Dependent edema
2. Jugular venous distention
3. Hepatojugular reflux and ascites
4. Atrial fibrillation
5. Cyanosis

What is the pathophysiologic basis of systolic dysfunction?

Decreased contractility

What are the two common causes of systolic dysfunction?

Ischemic cardiomyopathy and myocarditis

What is the pathophysiologic basis of diastolic dysfunction?

Decreased ventricular compliance

What are the four common causes of diastolic dysfunction?

1. HTN
2. Ischemic cardiomyopathy
3. Hypertrophic cardiomyopathy
4. Systemic disorders (i.e., amyloidosis, hemochromatosis)

Name four common chest x-ray (CXR) abnormalities in CHF.

1. Cardiomegaly
2. Cephalization of pulmonary vessels
3. Kerley B lines
4. Pleural effusions

Name two common echocardiographic abnormalities in CHF.

1. Decreased ejection fraction
2. Cardiomegaly

Name the CHF drug associated with each of the following statements:

Shown to decrease mortality in CHF	ACE inhibitors, β-blockers and spironolactone ($\downarrow$ mortality in class IV CHF)
Used acutely for worsening dyspnea and fluid retention	Loop diuretics
Reduces afterload by causing vasodilation of both arteries and veins	ACE inhibitors
Reduce symptoms of CHF by improving contractility	Digitalis
Vasodilators used in patients refractory to ACE inhibitors	Hydralazine and isosorbide dinitrate
May cause arrhythmias, yellow-tinted vision, anorexia, and nausea	Digitalis
Intravenous positive inotropic agents	Dopamine, dobutamine, and nesiritide

Valvular Heart Disease

Name the valvular defect associated with each of the following murmurs:

Harsh midsystolic murmur in the right second intercostal space at the right sternal border, radiating into the neck and apex	Aortic stenosis
Blowing, high-pitched diastolic murmur at left two to fourth interspaces radiating to apex	Aortic regurgitation
Blowing holosystolic murmur at apex radiating into left axilla with increased apical impulse	Mitral regurgitation
Low-pitched diastolic murmur at the apex that gets louder prior to S1; an opening snap is often present just after S2	Mitral stenosis
Soft, late systolic murmur at left sternal border or apex, accompanied by midsystolic click	Mitral valve prolapse
Harsh midsystolic murmur in the left second intercostal space at the left sternal border	Pulmonic stenosis

Blowing holosystolic murmur at lower left sternal border radiating to right of sternum; may increase with inspiration	Tricuspid regurgitation
Harsh holosystolic murmur at lower left sternal border, accompanied by thrill	Ventricular septal defect
Harsh midsystolic murmur in the third and fourth left interspaces radiating down left sternal border. S4 and biphasic apical impulse often present	Hypertrophic cardiomyopathy

Note: The above valvular diseases arranged in order of incidence.

Name the valvular defect associated with the following features:

Can be caused by papillary muscle rupture 2° to MI	Mitral regurgitation
May cause left atrial enlargement, atrial fibrillation, and pulmonary edema	Mitral stenosis and mitral regurgitation
Presents with triad of angina, syncope, and exertional dyspnea; boot-shaped heart on CXR	Aortic stenosis
May be precipitated by infective endocarditis, aortic aneurysmal dilation, and connective tissue disorders	Aortic insufficiency
Atrioventricular block	Mitral regurgitation
Calcific degeneration of a congenital bicuspid valve	Aortic stenosis
Increased pulse pressure	Aortic insufficiency

Cardiomyopathies

What are the most common etiologies of dilated cardiomyopathy?	**ABCDE**
	Alcohol abuse
	Beriberi
	Coxsackie B myocarditis, cocaine, Chagas disease
	Doxorubicin toxicity
	(Also: Pregnancy)

Name the type of cardiomyopathy associated with the following clinical features:

Asymmetric septal hypertrophy, banana-shaped left ventricle (LV); LV outflow obstruction	Hypertrophic
May be caused by sarcoidosis, amyloidosis, scleroderma, hereditary hemochromatosis, endocardial fibroelastosis, radiation induced fibrosis	Restrictive
Causes sudden death in young, otherwise healthy athletes	Hypertrophic
Four-chamber hypertrophy and dilation accompanied by systolic dysfunction	Dilated
Cardiomyopathy most commonly caused by endomyocardial fibrosis	Restrictive
Most common type of cardiomyopathy, commonly inherited in autosomal-dominant (AD) fashion	Hypertrophic
ACEi have been demonstrated to decrease mortality	Dilated
Symptoms relieved by squatting	Hypertrophic
Impaired left ventricular diastolic filling; may mimic constrictive pericarditis	Restrictive
Examination reveals cardiomegaly, mitral regurgitation, and S3; balloon-shaped heart on CXR	Dilated
Mitral regurgitation, sustained apical impulse, S4, and systolic ejection murmur; boot-shaped heart on CXR	Hypertrophic
β-Blockers and Ca^{2+} blockers provide symptomatic relief	Hypertrophic

Pericardial Disease

What is the common presentation of pericarditis?	Pleuritic retrosternal chest pain ($\uparrow$ when supine, $\downarrow$ when sitting up and leaning forward), dyspnea, cough, and fever

What are the most common etiologies of serous pericarditis?	Uremia, systemic lupus erythematosus (SLE), rheumatic fever, coxsackie viral infection
What are the most common etiologies of fibrinous pericarditis?	Uremia, SLE, rheumatic fever, coxsackie viral infection, MI
What are the most common etiologies of hemorrhagic pericarditis?	Trauma, malignancy, tuberculosis
What is a typical examination finding in pericarditis?	Pericardial friction rub
What are the classic ECG findings in pericarditis?	Diffuse ST elevation
What life-threatening complication of pericarditis causes distant heart sounds, jugular venous distention, hypotension, pulsus paradoxus, and elevated central venous pressure (CVP) on inspiration?	Cardiac tamponade
What is the definitive treatment for acute decompensation in a patient with cardiac tamponade?	Pericardiocentesis
What 2° intervention may be helpful in the management of a patient with cardiac tamponade?	Intravascular volume expansion

Endocarditis

What are the three major categories of endocarditis?	1. Infective 2. Nonbacterial thrombotic or marantic 3. Libman-Sacks endocarditis
What is the common presentation of infective endocarditis (IE)?	Fever (high in acute endocarditis, low-grade in subacute endocarditis), constitutional symptoms, and dyspnea
What are the clinical signs of IE?	**"JR NO FAME"** Janeway lesions Roth's spots Nail bed hemorrhages Osler's nodes Fever Anemia Murmur Emboli

What criteria are typically used for diagnosing IE?	The Duke criteria
What are the two major Duke criteria?	1. Two consecutive blood cultures (12 h apart) positive for IE-causing organism 2. Echocardiogram demonstrating valvular vegetation, ring abscess, or other evidence of endocardial infection
What are the six minor Duke criteria?	1. Cardiac predisposition including valvular abnormality, congenital heart disease, or hypertrophic cardiomyopathy 2. Fever >38°C 3. Signs of embolic disease including septic pulmonary emboli, mycotic cerebral abscesses, Janeway lesions 4. Immunologic phenomena including Roth's spots or Osler's nodes 5. Single positive blood culture 6. Echocardiographic findings consistent with but not diagnostic for endocarditis
What is the most common valve affected by IE?	Mitral valve
What is the most common valve affected by IE in IV drug users?	Tricuspid valve
Name the type of endocarditis described in each of the following clinical scenarios:	
25 y/o IV drug user with rapid onset of high fever, rigors, malaise with tricuspid regurgitation	Acute IE
60 y/o female with mitral valve prolapse who has recently undergone dental extraction presenting with low-grade fever and flu-like symptoms	Subacute IE
65 y/o male with metastatic colon cancer and a new murmur consistent with mitral regurgitation	Nonbacterial thrombotic endocarditis
30 y/o female with SLE	Libman-Sacks endocarditis
Which organism most often causes *acute* IE?	*Staphylococcus aureus*

Which organism most often causes *subacute* IE?

Streptococcus viridans

Which organisms can cause endocarditis but are not typically isolated by conventional bacterial culture?

HACEK organisms *(Haemophilus parainfluenzae, Actinobacillus, Cardiobacterium, Eikenella, Kingella)*

What are some sequelae of bacterial endocarditis?

Valvular injury, renal injury (glomerulonephritis [GN]), septic emboli to brain/lungs/kidneys causing infarction or abscess

What is the most common cause of myocarditis worldwide?

Trypanosoma cruzii (Chagas disease)

What is the empiric treatment for a patient with suspected endocarditis (before an organism is isolated in blood cultures)?

An antistaphylococcal β-lactam antibiotic and an aminoglycoside

What is the suggested regimen of antibiotic prophylaxis for patients at increased risk of endocarditis?

Two grams of amoxicillin prior to dental procedures

Rheumatic Heart Disease

What type of infection causes rheumatic fever?

Group A streptococcal pharyngitis

How does streptococcal pharyngitis cause rheumatic heart disease?

Antistreptococcal antibodies cross-react with a cardiac antigen

What serologic test is elevated in rheumatic heart disease?

Antistreptolysin antibodies (ASO), DNAse B

Name the five major Jones criteria for rheumatic heart disease.

"JONES"

Joints (migratory polyarthritis)

♥: pancarditis

N: subcutaneous nodules

Erythema marginatum

Sydenham's chorea

Name three minor Jones criteria for rheumatic heart disease.

1. Fever
2. Arthralgia
3. Leukocytosis

What is the most commonly observed valvular deformity in rheumatic heart disease?

Mitral stenosis

What treatment for streptococcal pharyngitis can prevent rheumatic heart disease?

Penicillin

What is the critical determinant of morbidity in acute rheumatic fever?	Degree of mitral and aortic valve stenosis/regurgitation

Aortic Dissection

What is the typical presentation of an aortic dissection?	Sudden onset severe, tearing substernal pain radiating to the interscapular region of the back
What PE findings are characteristic of an aortic dissection?	Unequal BP in the extremities, new murmur consistent with aortic regurgitation
What finding on CXR suggests an aortic dissection?	Widened mediastinum
What is the gold standard for the diagnosis of aortic dissection?	Angiography; (CT with contrast and MRI also have diagnostic use and are less invasive.)
What medication is preferred for lowering BP in a patient with an aortic dissection?	Sodium nitroprusside and β-blockers
What is the definitive therapy for an aortic dissection?	Surgical repair

Peripheral Vascular Disease (PVD)

What are the risk factors for PVD?	Similar to coronary risk factors; though diabetes is #1
Name the PVD associated with the following features:	
Focal neurologic findings	Cerebrovascular disease
Abdominal pain out of proportion to examination	Mesenteric ischemia
Intermittent claudication	Chronic arterial occlusive disease
Pain in buttocks and thighs with walking	Aortoiliac occlusive disease
Pain in calves with walking	Femoral-popliteal occlusive disease
Abdominal angina	Chronic mesenteric arterial occlusive disease
What noninvasive study is used to diagnose arterial occlusion?	Doppler ultrasound

What is the gold standard for the diagnosis of arterial occlusion? — Angiography

What is the source of most emboli causing acute arterial occlusion? — Cardiac mural thrombus (commonly in patients with atrial fibrillation)

What is the treatment of an acute arterial occlusion? — Surgical or percutaneous thrombectomy or medical thrombolysis

What type of therapy must be administered to all patients with a h/o acute arterial occlusion? — Warfarin

Make the Diagnosis

56 y/o female presents with dyspnea on exertion (DOE); PE: loud S1, delayed P2, early diastolic sound, and a diastolic rumble; Transesophageal echocardiogram: mobile, pedunculated left atrial mass — Atrial myxoma

60 y/o presents with chest pain relieved by sitting up and leaning forward; PE: pericardial friction rub; ECG: diffuse ST segment elevation; echocardiogram: pericardial effusion with thickening of the pericardium — Acute pericarditis

65 y/o male presents with 1 week h/o fever and DOE and orthopnea; PE: new blowing holosystolic murmur at apex radiating into left axilla; blood cultures ⊕ for viridans streptococci; echo: oscillating mass attached to mitral valve — Acute IE

60 y/o presents with dyspnea and palpitations; PE: 20 mmHg decline in systolic BP with inspiration (pulsus paradoxus), ↓ BP, JVD, diminished S1 and S2; echo: large pericardial effusion — Tamponade

58 y/o male with Marfan's syndrome presents with the abrupt onset of tearing chest pain radiating to the back; PE: ↓ BP, asymmetric pulses, declining mental status; CXR: widened mediastinum — Aortic dissection

70 y/o diabetic with hypercholesterolemia presents with angina, syncope, DOE; PE: diminished, slowly rising carotid pulses, crescendo-decrescendo systolic murmur at the second interspace at the right upper sternal border	Aortic stenosis
80 y/o diabetic with HTN and a h/o rheumatic heart disease presents with left-sided weakness; PE: pulses are irregularly irregular; ECG: absence of P waves and irregularly irregular QRS complexes	Atrial fibrillation (leading to embolic stroke)
70 y/o with a h/o CAD presents with worsening DOE, orthopnea, and paroxysmal nocturnal dyspnea; PE: JVD, S3 gallop, ⊕ hepatojugular reflex, bibasilar rales, and peripheral edema; CXR: cardiomegaly, bilateral pleural effusions	CHF
50 y/o chronic alcoholic presents with worsening DOE, orthopnea, and paroxysmal nocturnal dyspnea; PE: laterally displaced apical impulse; echocardiogram: four-chamber dilation, mitral and tricuspid regurgitation	Alcoholic dilated cardiomyopathy
35 y/o male with FH of sudden cardiac death presents with DOE and syncope; PE: double apical impulse, S4 gallop, holosystolic murmur at apex and axilla; echo: left ventricular hypertrophy and mitral regurgitation	Hypertrophic cardiomyopathy
40 y/o Black male with h/o HTN presents with chest pain, dyspnea, and severe headache; PE: BP = 210/130 in all four extremities, flame-shaped retinal hemorrhages, papilledema; labs: negative VMA and urine catecholamines, and cardiac enzymes	Malignant HTN
35 y/o female with a h/o rheumatic fever presents with worsening DOE and orthopnea; PE: loud S1, opening snap, and low-pitched diastolic murmur ' the apex; CXR: left atrial enlargement	Mitral stenosis

65 y/o male presents with 1 h h/o   Anterior MI
substernal pressure and pain with
radiation into the jaw and left arm,
nausea, and diaphoresis; PE: S4 gallop;
labs: ↑ troponin and CK-MB; ECG:
ST elevation in leads aVL, V1–V4

PULMONARY

Chronic Obstructive Pulmonary Disease (COPD)

Name the type of obstructive pulmonary
disease associated with the following
features:

Productive cough on most days during 3 or more consecutive months for 2 or more years that is worst in winter	Chronic bronchitis
Dyspnea and resultant hypertrophy of accessory muscles of inspiration	Emphysema
Cyanosis, rhonchi, wheezes, obesity, and signs of right-sided heart failure	Chronic bronchitis
Normal PaCO$_2$, mildly ↓ PO$_2$	Emphysema
Hypertrophy/hyperplasia of mucus glands lining the airways	Chronic bronchitis
Destruction of alveolar walls leading to loss of elastic recoil and dilation of airspaces	Emphysema
Acute or subacute onset of dyspnea, expiratory wheezing, prolonged expiratory phase, accessory muscle use	Asthma
Pursed-lip breathing, prolonged expiratory phase	Emphysema
Commonly caused by cystic fibrosis (CF), severe/chronic pulmonary infection, or connective tissue disease	Bronchiectasis
Mucous plugging, airway smooth muscle hypertrophy, peripheral eosinophilia	Asthma

Barrel chest, $\downarrow$ breath sounds, hyperresonant to percussion	Emphysema
$\uparrow PaCO_2$, $\downarrow PO_2$, $\uparrow$ hematocrit (Hct) early in the course of disease	Chronic bronchitis
Lung hyperinflation on CXR	Emphysema, asthma
Airway irritability causing reversible bronchoconstriction; diagnose with methacholine challenge	Asthma
Permanent dilation of bronchioles	Bronchiectasis
Mildly $\downarrow PaO_2$, respiratory alkalosis	Asthma
Halitosis, hemoptysis, and productive cough	Bronchiectasis
CXR may demonstrate subpleural blebs or parenchymal bullae	Emphysema
Exacerbation may be triggered by cold air, exercise, inhaled dust, upper respiratory infection (URI), β-blockers, stress	Asthma
CXR may show tram-track lung markings	Bronchiectasis
What is the most beneficial lifestyle modification for a patient with COPD?	Smoking cessation
What prophylactic vaccines are recommended for patients with COPD?	Influenza and pneumococcal vaccines
What are the three classes of bronchodilators used for COPD and asthma?	1. β_2-selective agonists 2. Anticholinergics 3. Methylxanthine
What bronchodilator commonly used in COPD for relief of nocturnal symptoms can also cause nausea, vomiting, seizures, and arrhythmias?	Theophylline
What two classes of drugs are useful during acute COPD exacerbations?	Corticosteroids and antibiotics
Which therapy can provide symptomatic relief and improve outcome in COPD patients with hypoxemia?	Supplemental oxygen therapy
What inherited disorder causes early progression of COPD?	α_1-Antitrypsin deficiency

Name the treatment of choice for the
following clinical scenarios in an asthmatic:

First-line therapy for acute asthmatic attack	O_2, bronchodilators, steroids
Second-line therapy for acute astmatic attack	$MgSO_4$ and intramuscular epinephrine
Initial therapy of mild asthma	Inhaled albuterol as needed
Mild asthma refractory to albuterol treatments	Inhaled glucocorticoids
Asthma attacks refractory to daily albuterol use	Systemic steroid therapy; usually with oral prednisone or IV methylprednisolone
Prophylaxis for asthma attacks (not including steroids)	Leukotriene inhibitors and cromolyn
Describe how glucocorticoids act on airways to control asthma.	↓ Inflammation and ↓ reactivity of airways to irritants (e.g., cold, cigarette smoke, allergens, exercise)

Restrictive Lung Disease

Name the specific type of lung disease
described below:

65 y/o hay farmer with recent exposure to moldy hay presents with chronic dry cough, chest tightness; PE: bilateral diffuse rales; bronchoscopy: interstitial inflammation; bronchioalveolar lavage: lymphocyte and mast cell predominance	Hypersensitivity pneumonitis
35 y/o male presents with intermittent hemoptysis and hematuria; W/U: alveolar hemorrhage and acute GN	Goodpasture's syndrome
40 y/o with progressive hypoxemia and cor pulmonale; lung biopsy: chronic inflammation of the alveolar wall in a pattern consistent with honeycomb lung, bronchioalveolar lavage: mild eosinophilia	Idiopathic pulmonary fibrosis
58 y/o former shipbuilder presents with the insidious onset of dyspnea; transbronchial biopsy demonstrates interstitial pulmonary fibrosis, ferruginous bodies; chest CT: demonstrates pleural effusion, and dense pleural fibrocalcific plaques	Asbestosis

55 y/o miner (nonsmoker) with dyspnea and dry cough; PFTs: obstructive and restrictive pattern; CXR: hilar lymphadenopathy with eggshell calcifications	Silicosis
60 y/o male with 100 pack-year h/o smoking presents with pleuritic chest pain, hemoptysis, and dyspnea; PE: dullness to percussion and absent breath sounds in the right lower lung field	Pleural effusion ($2°$ to malignancy)
50 y/o former heavy smoker presents with multiple lung and rib lesions; Excisional biopsy: lesions composed of cells (similar to the Langerhans cells of the skin) containing tennis racket-shaped Birbeck granules	Eosinophilic granuloma
30 y/o Black female presents with DOE, fever, arthralgia; PE: iritis, erythema nodosum; labs: eosinophilia, ↑ serum ACE levels; PFT: restrictive pattern; CXR: bilateral hilar lymphadenopathy; lymph node biopsy: noncaseating granulomas	Sarcoidosis

Cystic Fibrosis

What are the common presenting symptoms of an infant with CF?	Meconium ileus, diarrhea, steatorrhea, malabsorption, failure to thrive, prolonged jaundice, recurrent URIs
What are the common presenting signs on examination of an infant with CF?	Cyanosis, clubbing, hyperresonant lung fields with occasional crackles, rectal prolapse, abdominal distention
What is the traditional diagnostic test for CF?	Sweat chloride test (⊕ if >60 mEq/L)
What is the definitive test for CF?	Genetic analysis
Which drugs are known to be beneficial in the management of CF?	Bronchodilators, antibiotics, and anti-inflammatory agents
What dietary supplements are necessary for patients with CF?	Pancreatic enzyme supplements and vitamins A, D, E, and K (the fat-soluble vitamins)
What two methods are used to clear excess pulmonary secretions?	Physical therapy and DNAse therapy

Describe the effect of CF on each of the following organs:

Lungs	Recurrent pulmonary infections, bronchiesctasis. ↑ Resudual Volume (RV) and TLC in chronic disease; ↓ Forced Expiratory Volume in the first second (FEV_1)/FVC in acute exacerbation; pulmonary hemorrhage may occur
Pancreas	Variable defects in pancreatic exocrine function; may cause pancreatic insufficiency
Intestines	Mucus plugs → small bowel obstruction; meconium ileus in some infants
Salivary glands	Ductal dilation; squamous metaplasia of ductal epithelium and glandular atrophy
Liver	Plugging of bile cannaliculi → cirrhosis
Epididymis and ductus deferens	Obstruction → azospermia and infertility

What is the classic finding on pulmonary examination in a patient with idiopathic pulmonary fibrosis?

Fine expiratory crackles (*velcro crackles*)

How does interstitial lung disease affect alveolar gas diffusion and lung volumes?

Interstitial fibrosis decreases gas diffusion and lung volumes

Which group of interstitial lung diseases can present with a combination of obstructive and restrictive pattern on PFTs?

Pneumoconioses

Which group of interstitial lung diseases is caused by a deposition of immune complexes in the alveoli and granuloma formation?

Hypersensitivity pneumonitis

Name several commonly used drugs that are known to cause interstitial lung disease.

Bleomycin, vincristine, alkylating agents, and amiodarone

What are typical findings on CXR in a patient with interstitial lung disease?

Reticular or reticulonodular infiltrates or honeycomb lung

**Name the interstitial lung disease(s)
with the following findings on CXR:**

Bilateral linear opacities and broad pleural plaques	Asbestosis
Nodular opacities in the upper lung zones	Coal worker's pneumoconiosis, silicosis
Diffuse infiltrates in the upper lung zones	Berylliosis, hypersensitivity pneumonitis

Patients with silicosis are at increased risk for which infectious disease?	Tuberculosis
What is the definitive diagnostic test for interstitial lung diseases?	Biopsy
What are the two general principles of treatment for hypersensitivity pneumonitis and the pneumoconioses?	Corticosteroids and prevention of exposure to offending agent
What is the mainstay of treatment for patients with sarcoidosis?	Corticosteroids

Pleural Effusion

**Name the type of pleural effusion
(transudate, exudate, or both)
associated with the following features:**

Common presentation includes dyspnea, pleuritic chest pain, hemoptysis, cough	Both
Pathophysiologic mechanism is based on a breakdown of the pleural membrane and capillaries	Exudate
Due to excess production or inadequate reabsorption of pleural fluid	Both
Pathophysiologic mechanism is based on changes in Starling's forces	Transudate
Decreased breath sounds, tactile fremitus, and dullness to percussion in the region of the effusion	Both
Effusion containing bacteria	Exudate
Commonly caused by cirrhosis, nephrotic syndrome, protein losing enteropathy, or heart failure	Transudate

Commonly caused by malignancy, tuberculosis, infection, SLE, rheumatoid arthritis (RA)	Exudate
May be caused by a PE	Both
pH <7.2, glucose <50	Exudate
(Pleural lactate dehydrogenase [LDH])/(serum LDH) >0.6	Exudate
(Pleural protein)/(serum protein) <0.5	Transudate
Specific gravity of effusion >1.015	Exudate
Name three conditions which may lead to a pleural effusion containing amylase?	Pancreatitis, esophageal rupture (traumatic or postoperative), and malignancy
What term is used to describe an exudative pulmonary effusion which contains gross pus, has readily visible bacteria, has a glucose <50, or a pH <7?	Empyema (complicated parapneumonic effusion)
What type of analysis should be performed on a patient in which malignancy is thought to be the cause of a pleural effusion?	Cytology
What class of drugs is often used to treat a transudative effusion?	Diuretics
What procedure is performed to prevent reaccumulation of a malignant pleural effusion?	Pleurodesis
In addition to antibiotic coverage for pneumonia, what is the appropriate management for an empyema?	Chest tube drainage

Pulmonary Embolism

What is the incidence of PE in autopsies?	Greater than 50%
What is the incidence of PE in hospitalized patients?	20–25%
What is the etiology of 95% of pulmonary emboli?	Dislodged lower extremity deep venous thromboses (DVT)
What is the most common clinical presentation of PE?	Sinus tachycardia
What are the other common presenting symptoms of PE?	Fever, pleuritic chest pain, cough, dyspnea/tachypnea, swollen and painful leg, anxiety

What factors favor the development of a DVT?	Virchow's triad: 1. Stasis 2. Hypercoagulability 3. Endothelial dysfunction
What are the two most common CXR findings in a patient with PE?	1. Normal CXR 2. Cardiomegaly
What are the *classic* CXR findings in a patient with a PE?	Pleural effusion, Hampton's hump (a distal wedge-shaped infarct), Westermark's sign (hyperlucency in the region of lung supplied by the infarcted artery)
What is the most common ECG finding in a patient with PE?	Sinus tachycardia
What is the classic ECG finding in a patient with PE?	S1Q3T3 (S wave in lead I, Q wave and *inverted* T in lead III)
What two diagnostic tests are commonly used to diagnose PE?	Chest CT with contrast and ventilation/perfusion scan (when contrast is contraindicated)
What is the gold standard test for diagnosis of PE?	Pulmonary angiogram
What serologic test can assist in ruling out PE when negative?	D-dimer
What thrombolytic drug may be used in massive PE causing hemodynamic instability?	t-PA
What therapy is indicated for high-risk patients during the W/U of PE and for patients diagnosed with PE?	IV heparin
What are the contraindications for anticoagulation with heparin?	1. H/o heparin induced thrombocytopenia (HITS) 2. Intracranial hemorrhage or neoplasm 3. Recent major surgery 4. Bleeding diathesis
Why should heparin be continued for several days after warfarin therapy is begun?	1. Warfarin takes several days to become therapeutic 2. Initially warfarin induces a hypercoagulable state (by inactivating proteins C and S) which may cause skin necrosis
What methods are used for long-term prophylaxis for patients at risk of developing DVT?	Warfarin or IVC filter

What is an alternative to warfarin for outpatient DVT prophylaxis?	Low-molecular-weight heparin
What type of tumors commonly cause a DVT by inducing a hypercoagulable state?	Adenocarcinomas
What commonly used medication increases the risk of DVT?	Oral contraceptives
What is the most common genetic disease that predisposes to the development of DVT?	Factor V Leiden

Pulmonary Edema

What syndrome is suggested by the presence of acute, refractory hypoxemia, decreased lung compliance, and pulmonary edema in a patient with normal pulmonary capillary wedge pressure?	Acute respiratory distress syndrome (ARDS)
What syndrome is suggested by the presence of pulmonary edema in a patient with an elevated pulmonary capillary wedge pressure?	Cardiogenic pulmonary edema
What are the diagnostic criteria for ARDS?	1. Acute onset of respiratory distress 2. $PaO_2 : FiO_2$ ratio ≤ 200 3. Bilateral pulmonary infiltrates on CXR 4. Normal capillary wedge pressure
What is the most common risk factor for ARDS?	Sepsis
Name three additional common risk factors for ARDS.	Lung injury due to aspiration of gastric contents, trauma, pancreatitis, drug overdose, shock
What type of respiratory therapy is indicated in ARDS?	Mechanical ventilation

Pneumothorax (PTX)

What are the two most common presenting symptoms in spontaneous PTX?	Unilateral chest pain and dyspnea
What are the common presenting signs in a patient with spontaneous PTX?	Tachypnea, unilateral diminished/absent breath sounds, and hyperresonance to percussion

What is the most common cause of primary spontaneous PTX?	Rupture of subpleural apical bullae
What are the most common causes of 2° spontaneous PTX?	COPD (most common), CF, pulmonary infections (especially PCP pneumonia and TB), trauma, iatrogenic
What widely used ICU procedure carries the risk of PTX?	Placement of subclavian or internal jugular central venous catheters
What are the common presenting signs in a patient with tension PTX?	Dyspnea, tachypnea, jugular venous distention, hemodynamic instability
What is the appearance of a PTX on CXR?	Pleural stripe with absent lung markings
What are the classic findings on CXR in tension PTX?	Hyperlucent lung field (ipsilateral), depressed diaphragm (ipsilateral), tracheal and mediastinal deviation (away from PTX), and compression of the contralateral lung
What is the treatment of a spontaneous PTX?	**Asymptomatic** → observation and O_2 therapy; **symptomatic** → may require chest tube drainage
What is the management of a tension PTX?	Emergent needle thoracostomy at the second interspace at the midclavicular line

Pneumonia

What is the common presentation of typical (bacterial) pneumonia?	Fever >39°C, chills, cough productive of blood tinged, purulent sputum, pleuritic pain
What is the common presentation of atypical pneumonia?	Fever <39°C, nonproductive cough, headache, GI upset
What are the common physical findings in pneumonia?	Bronchial breath sounds, crackles, wheezes, egophany, dullness to percussion, and tactile fremitus
What is the classic CXR finding in typical pneumonia?	Lobar consolidation
What is the classic CXR finding in atypical pneumonia?	Patchy alveolar infiltrates

Name the most common organism(s) causing the pulmonary infection described below:

Lobar pneumonia

Streptococcus pneumoniae

Bronchopneumonia

S. aureus and *Haemophilus influenza*

Interstitial pneumonia

Mycoplasma pneumoniae (most common), *Legionella pneumophila, Chlamydia pneumonia*

Fungal pneumonia in AIDS patient with CD4$^+$ count <200

Pneumocystis carinii

Typical pneumonia in neonate

Streptococcus agalactiae

Alcoholic with typical pneumonia after aspiration

Klebsiella pneumoniae

Atypical pneumonia in younger patient with positive cold agglutinin test

M. pneumoniae

Neonate with atypical pneumonia and trachoma

C. trachomatis

Dairy worker with atypical pneumonia

Coxiella burnetti

Rabbit hunter with atypical pneumonia

Francisella tularensis

Pet bird owner with pneumonia, splenomegaly, bradycardia

Chlamydia psittaci

Hospitalized patient with lobar pneumonia

Streptococcus pneumoniae > Staphylococcus aureus

IV drug user with pneumonia

Streptococcus pneumoniae, Klebsiella pneumoniae, Staphylococcus aureus

Patient recovering from viral URI

S. aureus, H. influenza

Chicken farmer from the Ohio river valley with atypical pneumonia

Histoplasma capsulatum

Patient from southwestern United States with atypical pneumonia

Coccidioides immitis

Most common cause of community-acquired pneumonia

S. pneumoniae

Best treated with naficillin, oxacillin, methicillin, or vancomycin (for penicillin-resistant strains)

S. aureus

Causes severe pneumonia in CF patients and readily develops multidrug resistance

Pseudomonas spp.

Cough productive of dark red, currant jelly sputum production in an alcoholic or diabetic	*K. pneumoniae*
Rust-colored sputum	*S. pneumoniae*
Lobar pneumonia in a smoker with COPD; sputum with gram-negative rods and many leukocytes; best treated with macrolides	*H. influenzae*
Recommended treatment includes third generation cephalosporin or fluoroquinolone	Gram-negative rods: *Pseudomonas* spp., *K. pneumoniae, H. influenzae*
Pneumonia following influenza infection	*S. aureus*
Associated with inhalation of contaminated water droplets from air conditioners	*L. pneumophila*
Lung abscess with air/fluid level on CXR	*S. aureus*
Pneumonia accompanied by hyponatremia, mental status changes, diarrhea, and LDH >700	*L. pneumophila*
Gram positive, weakly acid-fast organism causing pneumonia in patients with AIDS; associated with peripheral eosinophilia	*Nocardia asteroides*
Fungus ball on CXR	*Aspergillus*

Name the most common causative pathogen(s) of pneumonia for each age group below:

Neonates	Group B streptococci, *Escherichia coli, C. pneumoniae*
Children (6 weeks to 18 years)	Respiratory syncytial virus (RSV) and other viruses, *M. pneumoniae, C. pneumoniae, S. pneumoniae*
Adults (18–40 years old)	*M. pneumoniae, C. pneumoniae, S. pneumoniae*
Adults (45–65 years old)	*S. pneumoniae, H. influenzae,* anaerobes, viruses, *M. pneumoniae*
Adults (>65 years old)	*S. pneumoniae,* viruses, anaerobes, *H. influenzae,* gram-negative rods

List the appropriate empiric therapy and most common organisms causing pneumonia in each of the following scenarios:

Community-acquired pneumonia in a healthy patient <60 y/o

Empiric therapy: macrolide, fluoroquinolone, or tetracycline

Organisms: *S. pneumoniae, M. pneumoniae, C. pneumoniae, H. influenzae,* and respiratory viruses

Community-acquired pneumonia in a healthy patient >60 y/o or with comorbidities (CHF, COPD, DM, alcoholic, renal or liver failure)

Empiric therapy: Second generation cephalosporin (e.g., cefuroxime) and amoxicillin; add erythromycin if atypical pathogens are suspected

Organisms: *Streptococcus pneumoniae, H. influenzae,* aerobic gram-negative bacilli, *Staphylococcus aureus,* and respiratory viruses

Community-acquired pneumonia in a patient requiring hospitalization

Empiric therapy: Antipneumococcal fluoroquinolone

Organisms: *S. pneumoniae* (including resistant strains), *H. influenzae, M. pneumoniae, C. pneumoniae,* polymicrobial

Community-acquired pneumonia in a patient requiring ICU admission

Empiric therapy: Antipseudomonal β-lactam (e.g., cefepime) plus an antipseudomonal quinolone (e.g., ciprofloxacin)

Organisms: *Streptococcus pneumoniae* (including resistant strains), *Legionella* spp., *H. influenzae,* enteric gram-negative bacilli, *Staphylococcus aureus,* and *P. aeruginosa*

Which patients should receive the pneumococcal vaccine?

Patients >65 y/o and immunocompromised patients (including postsplenectomy and sickle cell patients)

Name four common complications of lobar pneumonia.

1. Abscess formation (especially *S. aureus* and anaerobes)
2. Empyema or spread of infection to the pleural cavity
3. Organization of exudate to form scar tissue
4. Sepsis

What type of infection is characterized by localized suppurative necrosis of lung tissue?	Lung abscess
Name several bacterial pathogens capable of causing lung abscess.	*Staphylococci, streptococci*, gram-negative bacilli, anaerobes, oral flora
Name the two bacterial pathogens commonly associated with lobar pneumonia complicated by empyema.	*Streptococcus pneumoniae* > *Staphylococcus aureus*

Pulmonary Neoplasms

What is the most common cause of cancer deaths in the U.S. for both males and females?	Lung cancer
What is the most common type of malignant lung tumor?	Metastasic lesions
What are the most common primary lung tumors?	Adenocarcinoma and squamous cell carcinoma (equal incidence)
What are the common presenting symptoms of lung cancer?	Cough, hemoptysis, dyspnea, chest pain, constitutional symptoms
Name the type(s) of primary lung cancer associated with the following features:	
Central location	Squamous cell and small (oat) cell carcinomas
Peripheral location	Adenocarcinoma, large cell, and bronchioalveolar carcinoma
Commonly found within large bronchi	Squamous cell and small (oat) cell carcinomas
Clear link to smoking	Carcinoid
No clear link to smoking	Bronchoalveolar adenocarcinoma
Most malignant tumor (often metastatic at diagnosis)	Small (oat) cell carcinoma
Often secretes parathyroid hormone (PTH)-related peptide	Squamous cell carcinoma
Associated with production of ADH and ACTH	Small (oat) cell carcinoma
Carcinoembryonic antigen (CEA) ⊕	Adenocarcinoma

Secretion of 5-HT results in tachycardia, diarrhea, skin flushing, wheezing	Carcinoid
Tumor cells lining alveolar walls	Bronchioloalveolar adenocarcinoma
Giant pleomorphic cells, many cerebral metastasis, poor prognosis	Large cell
Associated with dermatomyositis, acanthosis nigricans	All types
Associated with peripheral neuropathy and Lambert-Eaton myasthenic syndrome	Small (oat) cell carcinoma
Associated with thrombophlebitis and marantic endocarditis	Adenocarcinoma

In each of the following clinical scenarios, name the structure being compressed or irritated by a lung tumor:

Cough	Phrenic nerve
Hoarseness	Recurrent laryngeal nerve
Facial and upper extremity swelling	Superior vena cava (SVC) syndrome
Ptosis, miosis, hemianhydrosis	Sympathetic cervical ganglion (Horner's syndrome)

What percentage of solitary pulmonary nodules are malignant?	40%
What is the differential diagnosis for a solitary pulmonary nodule?	Infectious granuloma, carcinoma, benign neoplasm, bronchial adenoma, pneumonia
Are routine CXRs a good way to screen for lung cancer/carcinoma (CA)?	No
What is an effective way to lower the risk of lung CA?	Smoking cessation
What is the treatment for small cell carcinoma?	Radiation and chemotherapy
What is the treatment for nonsmall cell carcinoma that is local?	Tumor resection and radiation therapy
What is the treatment for nonsmall cell carcinoma that has metastasized?	Radiation and chemotherapy
What rare pleural tumor is found in patients with a h/o occupational exposure to asbestos?	Malignant mesothelioma

owing features
y nodule favor
_t_ etiology:

	Malignant
	Malignant
We⎵ ⎵scribed mass	Benign
Absence of calcification or irregular calcification	Malignant
Growth in lesion from previous CXRs	Malignant
Central, uniform, or laminated calcification	Benign

Make the Diagnosis

7 y/o with h/o environmental allergies presents in acute respiratory distress; PE: ↑ tachypnea expiratory wheezes, intercostal retractions, accessory muscle use; CXR: hyperinflation; complete blood count (CBC) shows eosinophilia	Bronchial asthma
60 y/o with a 50 pack-year h/o smoking presents with fever and cough productive of thick sputum for the past 4 months; PE: cyanosis, crackles, wheezes; W/U: Hct = 48, WBC = 12,000, CXR: no infiltrates	Chronic bronchitis
60 y/o with a 50 pack-year h/o smoking presents with DOE and dry cough but no chest pain; PE: ↓ breath sounds, hyperresonant chest, ↑ heart rate (HR), distant S1 and S2; CXR: flattened diaphragm	Emphysema
60 y/o with 50 pack-year h/o smoking presents with fatigue, dyspnea, hoarseness, anorexia; PE: miosis, ptosis, anhydrosis, and dullness to percussion at right apex; Chest CT: large hilar mass extending into the right superior pulmonary sulcus	Pancoast tumor, (most likely bronchogenic squamous cell carcinoma, causing Horner's syndrome)

60 y/o patient is 4 days status post (s/p) total knee replacement has the sudden onset of tachycardia, tachypnea, sharp chest pain, hypotension; arterial blood gas (ABG): respiratory alkalosis; ECG: sinus tachycardia; Venous duplex ultrasound: clot in right femoral vein	Pulmonary embolus
40 y/o White male presents with chronic rhinosinusitis, ear pain, cough, dyspnea; PE: ulcerations of nasal mucosa, perforation of nasal septum; W/U: ↑ (C-ANCA), red cell casts in urine; Biopsy of nasal lesions: necrotizing vasculitis and granulomas	Wegener's granulomatosis

INFECTIOUS DISEASES

Fever

Name the six "do-not-miss" diagnoses of infections that present with fever and rash.	1. Meningococcemia 2. Bacterial sepsis (e.g., *Staphylococcus*) 3. Endocarditis 4. Gonococcemia 5. Rocky Mountain spotted fever (RMSF) 6. Typhoid fever
What criteria are used to define fever of unknown origin (FUO)?	Temperature >38.3°C (101°F) for >3 weeks with failure to diagnose (despite 1 week of inpatient investigation or several outpatient visits)
Name three common causes of FUO for each of the following categories:	
Infectious (30–40% of cases)	Endocarditis, TB, and occult abscess (usually abdominal)
Neoplastic (20–30% of cases)	Leukemia, lymphoma, and renal cell CA
Autoimmune (15–20% of cases)	Giant cell arteritis, polymyalgia rheumatica, and juvenile RA

Ear, Nose, and Throat Infections

Name four risk factors for sinusitis.	Smoking, viral infection, allergies, and barotrauma

What are the most common bacterial pathogens causing acute sinusitis?	*S. pneumoniae, H. influenzae, Moraxella catarrhalis*
What sinuses are most commonly involved in acute sinusitis?	Maxillary sinuses (drain superiorly against gravity)
Name three key clinical findings of acute sinusitis.	Purulent rhinorrhea, facial pain, maxillary tooth pain
What is the treatment of acute sinusitis lasting >2 weeks?	Bactrim or amoxicillin (10 days PO), decongestants
What condition results from obstruction of sinus drainage and ongoing anaerobic infection?	Chronic sinusitis
What is the treatment of chronic sinusitis?	6–12 weeks PO antibiotics; surgical correction of obstruction for refractory cases
Diabetics are at increased risk for developing what type of severe sinusitis?	Mucormycosis
Name four potential complications of sinusitis.	Meningitis, frontal bone osteomyelitis, abscess formation, and cavernous sinus thrombosis
Where do the majority of bleeds from epistaxis occur?	Kiesselbach's plexus (anterior nasal septum)
What is the most common cause of epistaxis in kids?	Exploration with digits
What are the two most common pathogens causing otitis externa (*swimmer's ear*)?	*Pseudomonas* and Enterobacteriaceae
What PE finding is virtually pathognomonic for otitis externa?	Pulling on pinna or pushing tragus causes pain
What is the treatment of choice for otitis externa?	Antibiotic eardrops (dicloxacillin for acute disease)
What group of patients is at ↑ risk for complications from otitis externa?	Diabetics—↑ risk of malignant otitis externa and osteomyelitis of temporal bone/skull base
Name the responsible organism and treatment for each of the following types of pharyngitis:	
Fever, sore throat, and red eye	Adenovirus
Oral thrush; seen in AIDS and small kids	Fungus (*Candida*)

Pathognomonic gray membranes on tonsils	Diphtheria (membranous pharyngitis)
High fever, sore throat with exudative tonsillitis, and cervical lymphadenopathy; cough usually absent	Group A streptococcus
Tonsillitis, splenomegaly, palatal petechiae, and posterior auricular lymphadenopathy	Epstein-Barr virus (EBV) (mononucleosis)

Tuberculosis (TB)

Decide whether each statement is more closely associated with 1° or 2° tuberculosis:

Classically affects lower lobes	Primary TB
Associated with reactivation	2° TB
Fibrocaseous cavitary lung lesion	2° TB
Ghon complex on CXR	Primary TB
Affects apical lungs (↑ affinity for ↑ O_2 environment)	2° TB
Presents with cough/hemoptysis, fever, night sweats, weight loss	2° TB

What is the primary mode of transmission of *Mycobacterium tuberculosis*?	Respiratory droplets
What term is used to describe the lymphatic and hematogenous spread of TB, causing numerous small foci of infection in extrapulmonary sites?	Miliary TB
Name the five most common sites of extrapulmonary TB.	1. CNS (tuberculous meningitis) 2. Vertebral bodies (Pott's disease) 3. Psoas major muscle → abscess 4. Liver 5. Cervical lymph nodes → scrofuloderma (massive lymphadenopathy)
How is active TB infection diagnosed?	Clinical and radiologic signs of 2° TB and acid-fast bacilli in sputum
What is an effective screening tool for latent TB?	Purified protein derivative (PPD) test

What constitutes a positive PPD test?	>5-mm induration for HIV⊕ or immunocompromised individuals >10-mm induration for high-risk individuals >15-mm induration for anyone else
What condition often causes a false negative PPD?	Immunosuppression → check anergy panel
What is the management of PPD ⊕ latent TB?	Treatment with isoniazid (INH) for 9 months
What is the management for active TB?	Respiratory isolation, initial four-drug therapy (INH, rifampin, ethambutol, pyrizinamide) → narrowed when sensitivities determined (treat for >6 months); **Note:** Give vitamin B_6 with INH
What is the major toxicity of many TB drugs?	Hepatotoxicity; check LFTs if symptomatic or h/o liver disease

Human Immunodeficiency Virus (HIV)

What test is used to rule out the diagnosis of HIV because of its high sensitivity?	Enzyme-linked immunosorbent assay (ELISA) (looks for antibody [AB] to viral proteins)
What test is used to confirm a positive HIV test because of its high specificity?	Western blot assay (high false negative within 2 months of infection)
What are the common presenting signs of the viral prodrome of HIV?	Constitutional symptoms (weight loss, fever, fatigue, night sweats) and/or neurologic symptoms (encephalopathy with dementia, aseptic meningitis)
How is AIDS defined?	$CD4^+$ <200 or serologic evidence of AIDS-defining illness
What mutation may confer resistance to infection with HIV?	Homozygous deletion of CCR5 (or other viral receptors)
Name the AIDS opportunistic infection or disease associated with the following:	
Fungal	*Candida* (thrush), *Cryptococcus* (meningitis), *P. carinii* pneumonia, histoplasmosis, coccidioidosis
Bacterial	*M. tuberculosis* (TB), *Staphylococcus*, encapsulated organisms, *M. avium-intracellulare* (MAC complex)

| Viral | Herpes simplex virus (HSV), varicella-zoster virus (VZV) (shingles), cytomegalovirus (CMV) (retinitis), JC virus (PML), Epstein-Barr virus (EBV) (B-cell lymphoma), human herpesvirus (HHV)-8 (Kaposi's sarcoma) |
| Protozoal | *Toxoplasma* (encephalopathy), *Cryptosporidium* (severe watery diarrhea) |

State the typical CD4$^+$ count associated with each of the following HIV complications:

Serious opportunists are first seen	<200 cells/mL
MAC, CMV, and cryptosporidiosis	<50 cells/mL
Toxoplasmosis, cryptococcosis	<100 cells/mL
TB becomes more common	<400 cells/mL

| What constitutes highly active antiretroviral therapy (HAART)? | Two nucleoside RT inhibitors combined with protease inhibitor or nonnucleoside RT inhibitor; **Note:** No patient should ever be on monotherapy due to the risk of resistance |

| What test is used to monitor the effectiveness of antiretroviral therapy? | HIV PCR (measures viral load) |

Name the medical management for the following HIV⊕ patients:

CD4$^+$ <500 or detectable viral load	Initiate HAART
CD4$^+$ <200	Bactrim prophylaxis for PCP
CD4$^+$ <75	Azithromycin prophylaxis for MAC
CD4$^+$ <50	Fluconazole prophylaxis for fungi
Pregnant HIV⊕ patient	Zidovudine (azidothymidine [AZT])—↓ vertical transmission

Urinary Tract Infections

Name six risk factors for urinary tract infection (UTIs).	1. Foley catheter
	2. Diabetes mellitus
	3. Anatomic anomaly
	4. Pregnancy
	5. ↑ Sexual activity
	6. H/o UTI or pyelonephritis

Name three common presenting symptoms in UTI.	Frequency, dysuria, and urgency
What two clinical findings suggest pyelonephritis?	Fever and back/flank pain
What is the most common presenting symptom in a child with a UTI?	Bedwetting
Why are women at 10× the risk of men for developing a UTI?	The urethra is shorter in women and more likely to be colonized with fecal flora

Name the specific urinary finding associated with each of the following:

Microscopic analysis in UTI	>5 WBC/high-power field
Urine dipstick in UTI	↑ Leukocyte esterace, ↑ nitrites
Clean-catch urine culture in a UTI	>100,000 CFU/mL of bacteria
Characteristic urinalysis (UA) finding in *Proteus* infection	↑ Urine pH
Characteristic UA finding in cystitis	Hematuria
Characteristic UA finding in acute pyelonephritis	WBC casts
List the most common UTI organisms.	**"SEEKS PP"**
	Serratia marcescens
	E. coli
	Enterobacter cloacae
	K. pneumoniae
	Staphylococcus saprophyticus
	Proteus mirabilis
	Pseudomonas aeruginosa
Which UTI-causing bug is frequently nosocomial, drug-resistant, and may produce a red pigment?	*S. marcescens*
What is the first-line antibiotic for lower UTIs?	Bactrim (trimethoprim [TMP]-sulfamethoxazole [SMX])

Sexually Transmitted Diseases

Name the sexually transmitted disease (STD) described below and provide the treatment of choice:

Clue cells in pap smear; positive "whiff test"	Bacterial vaginosis (e.g., *Gardnerella vaginitis*) **Tx** = Flagyl (metronidazole)
Soft, painful sexually transmitted ulcer associated with inguinal lymphadenopathy	Chancroid (caused by *Haemophilus ducreyi*) **Tx** = Ceftriaxone, ciprofloxacin, or erythromycin
Raised, red papules; biopsy shows Donovan bodies	Granuloma inguinale (caused by *Calymmatobacterium granulomatis*) **Tx** = doxycycline 100 mg bid × 3 weeks
Firm, painless chancre caused by a spirochete	Syphilis (caused by *Treponema pallidum*) **Tx** = Penicillin G
Most common STD; frequent cause of pelvic inflammatory disease (PID) in women and urethritis in men; associated with Reiter's syndrome	Chlamydial cervicitis (types D–K) **Tx** = azithromycin; erythromycin in pregnancy; treat presumptive gonorrhea coinfection
Small papule/ulcer that leads to enlargement of lymph nodes; caused by *C. trachomatis* serotypes L1, L2, or L3	Lymphogranuloma venereum **Tx** = same as above
STD that can result in extragenital infections (e.g., pharyngitis, proctitis, arthritis, and neonatal conjunctivitis)	Gonorrhea (caused by *Neisseria gonorrhoeae*) **Tx** = ceftriaxone; treat presumptive chlamydia coinfection
STD resulting in benign venereal warts caused by human papillomavirus (HPV) types 6 and 11	Condyloma acuminatum **Tx** = cryotherapy or topical podophyllin
Painful vesicles/ulcers; cytology shows multinuclear giant cells; diagnose with Tzanck prep	Herpes genitalis (most often HSV type 2) **Tx** = acyclovir (for $1°$ infection or suppression)
STD caused by flagellated, motile protozoan; #2 cause of vaginitis	Trichomoniasis **Tx** = flagyl (metronidazole)

Name the stage of syphilis associated
with each of the following
descriptions:

    Rash on palms and soles with $2°$ syphilis
    lymphadenopathy

    Firm, painless chancre $1°$ syphilis

    After 1 year of infection; can progress   Late latent
    to $3°$ syphilis

    1st year of infection; no symptoms,   Early latent
    but positive serology

    Tabes dorsalis, aortitis, Argyll- $3°$ syphilis
    Robertson pupil, gummas

Name three tests that can be used to
diagnose syphilis.

1. Dark-field microscopy (visible spirochetes)
2. VDRL/RPR (fast, cheap, nonspecific)
3. Fluorescent treponemal antibody—absorbed (FTA-ABS) (sensitive, specific, positive for life)

What is the treatment for syphilis?

Penicillin (IV for neurosyphilis); $\uparrow$ dose by 3× if undiagnosed for >1 year

What complication of syphilis treatment
results in fever and flu-like symptoms
caused by the massive destruction of
spirochetes?

Jarisch-Herxheimer reaction

Osteomyelitis

What are the two main routes of infection
for osteomyelitis?

Direct spread (80%) or hematogenous seeding (20%)

Where does hematogenous osteomyelitis
typically occur?

Metaphyses of long bones in children ($\uparrow$ vascularity of growth plates); vertebral bodies of IV drug abusers

Name the organism typically responsible
for osteomyelitis in each of the
following situations:

    Newborn   *Streptococci* spp. *or E. coli*

    Child   *Staphylococcus aureus*

Otherwise healthy adult	*S. aureus*
Foot puncture wound	*Pseudomonas* spp.
Intravenous drug user	*Pseudomonas* spp. *or S. aureus*
Sickle cell disease	*Salmonella* spp.
Hip replacement (or other prosthesis)	*Staphylococcus epidermidis*
Chronic osteomyelitis	*S. aureus, Pseudomonas* spp., *Enterobacteriaceae*
Asplenic patient	*Salmonella* spp.

What is the classic radiographic finding in osteomyelitis?	Periosteal elevation
What is the gold standard for evaluation of osteomyelitis?	MRI (can confirm with bone aspiration and culture)
What is the treatment regimen for pyogenic osteomyelitis?	6–8 weeks of antibiotics; fluoroquinolones empirically $\rightarrow$ narrow as cultures come back; surgical debridement if necessary
Name four complications of osteomyelitis?	1. Chronic osteomyelitis 2. Septic arthritis 3. Systemic sepsis 4. Draining sinus tract $\rightarrow$ squamous cell carcinoma

Vector-borne Illness

What is the most common vector-borne disease in the United States?	Lyme disease
Name the organism and the vector involved in Lyme disease.	*Borrelia burgdorferi* is carried by *Ixodes* ticks
What is the treatment for Lyme disease?	Ceftriaxone, high-dose penicillin, or doxycycline
Name the stage of Lyme disease associated with each of the following classic PE findings:	
Migratory polyarthropathy/arthralgias, meningitis, myocarditis (with conduction defects), neurologic problems	2° Lyme disease
Erythema chronicum migrans	Primary Lyme disease
Encephalitis and arthritis	Tertiary (3°) Lyme disease

What tick-borne disease can lead to small vessel vasculitis?	RMSF
Name the organism and the vector involved in RMSF.	*Rickettsia rickettsii* is carried by Dermacentor tick
Name four common PE findings in RMSF.	Fever, headache, myalgias, classic maculopapular rash (begins on palms/soles → spreads centrally)
What is the differential diagnosis for a rash affecting the palms and soles?	RMSF, 2° syphilis, hand-foot-mouth disease (coxsackie A), and Kawasaki syndrome
What is the treatment for RMSF?	Doxycycline; chloramphenicol in pregnant women and kids

Sepsis

What is sepsis?	An infection that causes systemic inflammatory response syndrome
What type of bacteria cause shock through endotoxin-mediated vasodilation?	Gram-negative bacteria

Name the organism(s) that most commonly cause sepsis in the following groups:

IV drug abusers	*S. aureus*
Asplenic/sickle cell patients	Encapsulated bacteria (*H. influenzae, Meningococcus, Pneumococcus*)
Neonates	Group B strep, *Klebsiella, E. coli*
Children	*H. influenzae, Meningococcus, Pneumococcus*
Adults	Gram-positive cocci, anaerobes, aerobic bacilli

State how each of the following parameters is affected in septic shock:

Temperature	↑ (though 15% present with hypothermia)
Respirations	↑
HR	↑
BP or total peripheral resistance (TPR)	↓
Cardiac output	↑
Pulmonary capillary wedge pressure	↓ (or sometimes normal)

What is the first-line management of septic shock?

Aggressive IV fluids, vasopressors, IV empiric antibiotics, removal of potential source (e.g., catheter, IV line)

Make the Diagnosis

18 y/o student returns to clinic with a rash after being treated with ampicillin for fever and sore throat; PE: tonsillar exudates and enlarged posterior cervical lymph nodes; labs: ↑ lymphocytes and ⊕ heterophil AB test

Infectious mononucleosis (EBV)

17 y/o swimmer presents with pain and discharge from the left ear; PE: movement of tragus is extremely painful

Otitis externa

2-month-old with maternal h/o rash and flu in first trimester presents with failure to attain milestones; PE: microcephaly, cataracts, jaundice, continuous machinery-like murmur at left upper sternal border (LUSB) and hepatosplenomegaly (HSM)

Congenital rubella

8 y/o from Connecticut presents with fever, rash, headache, and joint pain after playing in the woods; PE: distinctive macule with surrounding 6 cm target-shaped lesion

Lyme disease

Newborn with h/o IUGR presents with rash and maternal h/o "flu" during first trimester; PE: petechial rash, chorioretinitis, microcephaly, ↓ hearing, and HSM; CBC: thrombocytopenia; Head CT: periventricular calcifications

Congenital CMV

25 y/o West Virginian male presents with fever, headache, myalgia, and a petechial rash that began peripherally but now involves his whole body, even his palms and soles; ⊕ OX19 and OX2 Weil-Felix reaction

Rocky mountain spotted fever (RMSF)

28 y/o with h/o syphilis treatment (5 h ago) with IM penicillin presents with fever, chills, muscle pain, and headache

Jarisch-Herxheimer reaction

26 y/o sexually active, native-Caribbean presents with painless, beefy-red ulcers of the genitalia and inguinal swelling; Peripheral blood smear: Donovan bodies on Giemsa-stained smear

Granuloma inguinale

31 y/o obese female presents with pruritis in her skin fold beneath her pannus; PE: whitish-curd-like concretions beneath the abdominal pannus; W/U: budding yeast on 10% KOH prep

Cutaneous candidiasis

GASTROENTEROLOGY

Diarrhea

Name the four major pathophysiologic mechanisms for chronic diarrhea.

1. Increased secretion
2. Altered intestinal motility
3. Osmotic load
4. Inflammation

What two laboratory tests can be used to distinguish between osmotic and secretory diarrhea?

Fasting (persistent diarrhea if secretory) and stool osmotic gap (gap >50 → osmotic diarrhea)

What additional labs are useful in the W/U of osmotic diarrhea?

D-Xylose test, Schilling test (terminal ileum), lactose challenge, and pancreatic enzymes

What is the main cause of surreptitious diarrhea?

Mg^{2+} laxative overuse

Which syndrome is characterized by irregular bowel movements, abdominal pain, and comorbid psychiatric disorders (in 50% of cases)?

Irritable bowel syndrome

Name the food poisoning bacteria associated with the following:

    Reheated rice

Bacillus cereus

    Reheated meat dishes

Clostridium perfringens

    Improperly canned food

Clostridium botulinum

    Contaminated seafood or raw oysters

Vibrio parahaemolyticus and *Vibrio vulnificus*

    Meats, mayonnaise, custards

S. aureus

    Undercooked meats

E. coli O157:H7

    Raw poultry, milk, eggs, and meat

Salmonella

| Name six infectious causes of bloody diarrhea. | 1. *Salmonella*
2. *Shigella*
3. *Campylobacter jejuni*
4. Enteroinvasive and enterohemorrhagic *E. coli*
5. *Yersinia enterocolitica*
6. *Entamoeba histolytica* |

Name the diarrhea-causing organism associated with the following statements:

Most common cause of diarrhea in infants	Rotavirus
10–12 bloody and mucous diarrhea stools per day due to ingestion of cysts	*E. histolytica*
Comma-shaped organisms causing rice-water stools	*Vibrio cholera*
Second to rotavirus as a cause of gastroenteritis in kids	Adenovirus (serotypes 40 and 41)
Bloody diarrhea; very low ID_{50}; nonmotile	*Shigella*
Usually transmitted from pet feces	*Y. enterocolitica*
Motile; lactose nonfermenter; causes bloody diarrhea	*Salmonella*
Comma- or S-shaped organisms causing bloody diarrhea; associated with Guillain-Barré syndrome	*C. jejuni*
Watery diarrhea with extensive fluid loss in AIDS patient	*Cryptosporidium*
Foul-smelling diarrhea after returning from a camping trip	*Giardia lamblia*
Watery diarrhea cause by antibiotic-induced suppression of colonic flora	*Clostridium difficile*

Inflammatory Bowel Disease (IBD)

Ulcerative colitis (UC) or Crohn's disease?

Pancolitis with crypt abscesses	UC
Fistulas and fissures	Crohn's disease
Associated with ankylosing spondylitis	Both
Associated with sclerosing cholangitis	UC

Amyloidosis	Crohn's disease
Longitudinal ulcers	Crohn's disease
Punched-out aphthous ulcers	Crohn's disease
Can lead to toxic megacolon	UC
Increased risk of colorectal carcinoma	UC >>> Crohn's
Skip lesions	Crohn's disease
Can involve any portion of the GI tract (usually *terminal ileum* and colon)	Crohn's disease
"String sign" on x-ray (due to bowel wall thickening)	Crohn's disease
Associated with pyoderma gangreosum	Both
Transmural inflammation	Crohn's disease
Noncaseating granulomas	Crohns disease
Cobblestone mucosa	Crohn's disease
Bloody diarrhea	UC
Watery diarrhea	Crohn's disease
Nephrolithiasis	Crohns disease
Stricture formation	Crohn's disease
Psuedopolyps	UC
Rectal involvement	UC
May mimic acute appendicitis	Crohn's disease
What is the key component of a diagnostic W/U of a patient with suspected IBD?	Colonoscopy with mucosal biopsies
What additional radiologic tests are useful in the W/U of Crohn's disease?	Upper GI series and small bowel follow through
What are the five classes of medical treatment of (IBD) disease?	1. Immunosuppressive agents (6-MP, azathioprine, methotrexate, cyclosporine) 2. 5-ASA derivatives (mesalamine, sulfasalazine) 3. Steroids (helpful in acute disease and during exacerbations) 4. Antibiotics (metronidazole for anal disease) 5. Monoclonal antibodies to TNFα (infliximab)

What are the indications for surgery in a patient with Crohn's disease?

1. Intestinal obstruction (most common indication for surgery)
2. Anorectal abscesses
3. Abdominal abscesses (percutaneous drainage)
4. Fistulas
5. Intractable disease

What are the two options for operative management of an obstruction in Crohn's disease?

Bowel resection versus strictureplasty

What complication can occur in a patient with multiple bowel resections?

Short gut syndrome (diarrhea, malabsorption)

Is surgery usually curative for Crohn's disease?

No

What are the indications for surgery in a patient with UC?

1. Uncontrolled hemorrhage
2. Fulminant colitis
3. Toxic megacolon
4. Dysplasia or cancer
5. Intractable disease

What are the three classic signs and symptoms of toxic megacolon?

Fever, abdominal pain, and acutely distended colon

What is the *initial* treatment of toxic megacolon?

Nothing by mouth (NPO), IV fluids nasogastric (NGT), and antibiotics

What surgical options are commonly used in patients with refractory UC?

Total proctocolectomy, distal rectal mucosectomy, and ileonal pull through

What is the risk of colon cancer in patients with UC?

1–2% at 10 years; 1% increase in risk every year thereafter

What are the recommendations for colon cancer surveillance in patients with UC?

Yearly colonoscopy after 10 years of disease

Is surgery curative for UC involving the colon?

Yes

What extraintestinal manifestations of UC are cured by surgery?

Pathology of the skin, eyes, and joints

What extraintestinal manifestations of UC are made worse by surgery?

Liver disease

Liver

Name the viral hepatitis agent(s)
described by the following statements:

Fecal-oral transmission	Hepatitis A virus (HAV) and hepatitis E virus (HEV)
Infection leads to a carrier state	Hepatitis B virus (HBV), hepatitis C virus (HCV), and hepatitis D virus (HDV) delta agent
Defective virus requiring hepatitis B surface antigen (HBsAg) as its envelope	HDV (delta agent)
Sexual, parenteral, and transplacental transmission	HBV, HCV, HDV
High mortality rate in pregnant women	HEV
Most common cause of IV drug use hepatitis in the United States	HCV
Long incubation (~3 months)	HBV
Increased risk of hepatocellular carcinoma	HBV, HCV
Immune globulin vaccine available	HAV, HBV (and HDV)

Name the hepatitis serologic marker
described below:

Antigen found on surface of HBV; continued presence suggests carrier state	HBsAg
Antigen associated with core of HBV	Hepatitis B core antigen (HBcAg)
Antigen in the HBV core that indicates transmissibility	Hepatitis Be antigen (HBeAg)
AB suggesting low HBV transmissibility	Hepatitis Be antibody (HBeAb)
Acts as a marker for HBV infection during the "window" period	Hepatitis B core antibody (HBcAb) (IgM in acute stage)
Provides immunity to HBV	HBsAb

What is the "window" period of a hepatitis infection?	Period during acute infection when HBsAg has become undetectable, but HBsAb has not yet appeared
Name six common causes of cirrhosis.	1. Chronic alcoholism 2. Hereditary hemochromatosis 3. Primary biliary cirrhosis 4. Wilson's disease (hepatolenticular degeneration) 5. Viral (HBV, HCV) 6. α_1-Antitrypsin deficiency

List the effects of hepatic failure on the following body systems:

Ocular	Scleral icterus
Dermatologic	Jaundice, spider nevi
Reproductive	Testicular atrophy, gynecomastia, loss of pubic hair
Hematopoietic	Anemia, bleeding tendency ($\downarrow$ coagulation factors), pancytopenia
Neurologic	Coma, hepatic encephalopathy (asterixis, hyperreflexia, behavioral changes
Renal	Hepatorenal syndrome (acute renal failure [ARF] $2°$ to hypoperfusion)
GI	Esophageal varicies, peptic ulcer, hemorrhoids

Name the liver disorder associated with each of the following findings:

Mallory bodies	Alcoholic hepatitis
Occlusion of IVC or hepatic veins with centrilobular congestion → congestive liver disease; associated with polycythemia, pregnancy, and hepatocellular carcinoma.	Budd-Chiari syndrome
Viral infection and salicylates in kids	Reye's syndrome
Copper deposition in liver, kidney, brain, and cornea → asterixis, basal ganglia degeneration, dementia	Wilson's disease (hepatolenticular degeneration)
AST:ALT ratio >1.5	Alcoholic hepatitis
Microvesicular fatty change occurring with fatal childhood hepatoencephalopathy	Reye's syndrome

State the etiology of cirrhosis associated with the following clinical or pathologic findings:

Panacinar pulmonary emphysema	α_1 Antitrypsin deficiency
Decreased ceruloplasmin	Wilson's disease (hepatolenticular degeneration)
Triad of bronze diabetes, skin pigmentation, and micronodular pigment cirrhosis	Hereditary hemochromatosis

Antimitochondrial antibodies	Primary biliary cirrhosis
Kayser-Fleischer ring	Wilson's disease (hepatolenticular degeneration)
Micronodular fatty liver; portal HTN, asterixis, jaundice, and gynecomastia	Chronic alcohol abuse
↑ ferritin, transferrin, and total iron; ↓ total iron-binding capacity (TIBC)	Hereditary hemochromatosis; **Note:** Total body iron sometimes high enough to trigger metal detectors.
What test can be used to determine the etiology of ascites?	Paracentesis and serum-ascites albumin gradient (SAAG)
Name four etiologies of ascites with SAAG <1.1.	1. Malignancy 2. Tuberculosis 3. Pancreatitis 4. Nephrotic syndrome
Name five etiologies of ascites with SAAG >1.1.	1. Cirrhosis 2. Hepatic metastases 3. Budd-Chiari syndrome 4. Cardiac disease 5. Myxedema
What are the three medical therapeutic options for ascites?	Salt restriction, diuretics (spironolactone), large volume paracentesis, and peritoneovenous shunting
Name the three general etiologic categories of portal HTN?	1. *Perisinusoidal* (e.g., splenic/portal vein thrombosis, schistosomiasis) 2. *Sinusoidal* (cirrhosis → 90% of all causes) 3. *Postsinusoidal* (e.g., right heart failure, hepatic vein thrombosis, constrictive pericarditis)
Name five complications of portal HTN?	1. Ascites 2. Spontaneous bacterial peritonitis (SBP) 3. Hepatorenal syndrome 4. Hepatic encephalopathy 5. Esophageal varices
What must be present in ascitic fluid to make the diagnosis of SBP?	Absolute neutrophil count of >250 (in symptomatic patients), >500 (in asymptomatic patients), or ⊕ Gram stain

Name three clinical findings in portal HTN resulting from the portal-systemic collateral circulation.	Esophageal varices, caput medusa, and hemorrhoids
What is the diagnostic test for bleeding varices?	esophagogastroduodenoscopy (EGD)
What methods are used to control acute upper GI bleeding caused by a bleeding esophageal varix?	Endoscopic sclerotherapy, IV vasopressin, and balloon tamponade with Sengstaken-Blakemore tube
What is the main interventional procedure used to manage portal HTN?	Shunt procedure (e.g., transjugular intrahepatic portacaval shunt [TIPS])
What is the main complication of a shunt procedure?	Worsening of hepatic encephalopathy ($2°$ ↓ flow to liver)
What is the classification system used in cirrhosis?	Child's criteria (A, B, or C-worst)
What five criteria are used for classification in the Child's system?	Bilirubin, albumin, ascites, encephalopathy, and nutrition
Name two drugs used to treat hepatic encephalopathy.	Lactulose (↓ ammonia absorption) and neomycin (decreases ammonia production from GI tract)
What is the only definitive therapy for cirrhotic liver disease?	Liver transplant
What are the three absolute contraindications for liver transplantation?	1. Infection outside of hepatobiliary system (e.g., AIDS) 2. Metastatic liver disease 3. Uncorrectable coagulopathy

Make the Diagnosis

20 y/o female presents with bloody diarrhea and joint pain; PE: abdominal tenderness, guaiac ⊕ stool; labs: ↑ ESR and CRP, HLA-B27 ⊕ ; colonoscopy: granular, friable mucosa with pseudopolyps throughout the colon	Ulcerative colitis
28 y/o patient with h/o of UC presents with severe abdominal pain, distention, and high fever; PE: severe abdominal tenderness; CBC: leukocytosis; Abdominal x-ray (AXR): dilated (>6 cm) transverse colon	Toxic megacolon

A cirrhotic patient presents with massive hematemesis; PE: jaundice, ↓ BP, ↑ HR, ascites; CBC: pancytopenia; LFTs: ↑ ALT and AST; EGD: actively bleeding vessel with numerous cherry red spots	Esophageal varices
38 y/o male with recent h/o fatigue, excessive thirst, and impotence presents with hyperpigmentation of his skin; PE: cardiomegaly, HSM; W/U: ↑ glucose, ferritin, transferrin, and serum iron	Hemochromatosis (hereditary)
19 y/o female with recent h/o behavioral disturbance presents with jaundice and resting tremor; PE: pigmented granules in cornea and HSM; W/U: ↓ serum ceruloplasmin	Wilson's disease
29 y/o with h/o intermittent jaundice since receiving blood transfusion after motor vehicle accident (MVA) 2 years ago; PE: right upper quadrant (RUQ) tenderness, hepatomegaly; W/U: negative HBV serology	Hepatitis C infection
31 y/o female presents with 10-month h/o foul-smelling, greasy diarrhea; PE: pallor, hyperkeratosis, multiple ecchymoses, and abdominal distention; W/U: abnormal D-xylose test	Celiac disease
A patient with recent h/o antibiotic use for sinus infection presents with fever, bloody diarrhea, and abdominal pain; PE: tender abdominal examination, guaiac ⊕ stool; CBC: leukocytosis; Colonoscopy: tan nodules seen attached to erythematous bowel wall with superficial erosions	Pseudomembranous colitis (*C. difficile* colitis)
60 y/o White male presents with steatorrhea, weight loss, arthritis, and fever; small bowel biopsy shows PAS ⊕ macrophages and gram-positive bacilli	Whipple disease
A patient presents with sudden onset of severe watery diarrhea, vomiting, and abdominal discomfort 4 h after eating potato salad at a picnic; the symptoms resolve spontaneously within 24 h	*S. aureus*-induced diarrhea

23 y/o female with h/o depression presents with abdominal discomfort and irregular bowel habits; W/U: stool cultures, electrolytes, and imaging studies all WNL

Irritable bowel syndrome

A patient traveling in Mexico presents with bloody diarrhea, vomiting, and abdominal cramps 16 h after drinking tap water; PE: low-grade fever, abdominal pain; W/U: ova and parasites in stool

Entamoeba histolytica-induced diarrhea

19 y/o Jewish female with h/o chronic abdominal pain presents with recurrent UTIs and pneumaturia; PE: diffuse abdominal pain; CT: enterovesical fistula; Colonoscopy: skip lesions of linear ulcers and transverse fissures giving cobble-stone appearance to mucosa

Crohn's disease

RENAL/GENITOURINARY

Basic Metabolism and Electrolytes

How is the anion gap calculated?

$Na^+ - (Cl^- + HCO_3^-)$

What is a normal anion gap?

8–12 mEq/L

List four causes of nongap metabolic acidosis.

1. Diarrhea
2. Renal tubular acidosis (RTA)
3. Spironolactone
4. TPN

List nine possible causes of anion gap metabolic acidosis.

"MUD PILERS"

Methanol

Uremia

Diabetic Ketoacidosis (DKA)

Paraldehyde

INH or Iron tablet overdose

Lactic acidosis

Ethylene glycol or Ethanol

Rhabdomyolysis (massive)

Salicylate toxicity

List the most common mechanism of respiratory acidosis.	Hypoventilation; causes include lung obstruction (acute/chronic lung disease) and neuromuscular disorders (sedatives, weakening of respiratory muscles)
List four causes of respiratory alkalosis.	1. Hyperventilation ($2°$ to hypoxia) 2. Early ASA ingestion 3. Pregnancy 4. Cirrhosis
List four causes of chloride-responsive (*dry*) metabolic alkalosis.	1. Excessive vomiting 2. Villous adenoma 3. Diuretics 4. Contraction alkalosis.
List three diseases causing chloride-unresponsive (*wet*) metabolic alkalosis.	1. Cushing's syndrome 2. Conn's syndrome 3. Bartter syndrome
Ingestion of what substance can cause both a metabolic acidosis and respiratory alkalosis?	ASA (salicylates)

Name the primary acid/base disturbance and the compensatory response that has occurred:

pH >7.4, PCO_2 >40 mmHg	Metabolic alkalosis $\rightarrow$ hypoventilation
pH <7.4, PCO_2 >40 mmHg	Respiratory acidosis $\rightarrow$ renal HCO_3^- reabsorption
pH >7.4, PCO_2 <40 mmHg	Respiratory alkalosis $\rightarrow$ renal HCO_3^- secretion
pH <7.4, PCO_2 <40 mmHg	Metabolic acidosis $\rightarrow$ hyperventilation

Name the electrolyte imbalance associated with the following conditions:

Diabetes insipidus (DI) or osmotic diuresis	Hypernatremia
ARF, adrenal insufficiency, spironolactone, rhabdomyolysis, acidosis, insulin deficiency, and digitalis poisoning	Hyperkalemia
Syndrome of inappropriate antidiuretic hormone secretion (SIADH), volume depletion, water intoxication, cirrhosis, heart failure, and hyperglycemia	Hyponatremia

Diarrhea, alkalosis, hypomagnesemia, laxative abuse, RTA, vomiting, and Bartter syndrome	Hypokalemia
Acute pancreatitis, hypomagnesemia, post-parathyroidectomy (most common cause)	Hypocalcemia
Malnutrition, alcoholism, DKA, and pregnancy	Hypomagnesemia

Name the ECG changes associated with the following electrolyte imbalances:

Hyperkalemia	In order: 1. Peaked T waves 2. ↑ PR interval 3. Loss of P wave 4. Widened QRS complex 5. Sine wave
Hypokalemia	T-wave flattening, U waves, ST depression and AV block
Hypocalcemia	↑ QT interval
Hypomagnesemia	Torsades de pointes

Name the main causes of hypercalcemia.

"CHIMPANZEES"

Calcium supplementation

Hyperparathyroidism (most common)

Iatrogenic/Immobility

Milk alkali syndrome

Paget's disease

Neoplasm (very common)

Zollinger-Ellison (ZE) syndrome

Excess vitamin A

Excess vitamin D

Sarcoidosis

Provide the treatment for the following electrolyte disturbances:

Hypernatremia	Isotonic NS or LR (correct over a 48–72 h period)
Hyponatremia	If $Na^+ <120$ → hypertonic NS; if *hypovolemic* → isotonic NS (rapid ↑ in plasma Na^+ → **central pontine myelinolysis**); if *euvolemic or hypervolemic* → salt and water restriction

Hyperkalemia	"See big K^+ die" → "C BIG Kay Di"
	Calcium gluconate (stabilizes cardiac membrane)
	Bicarbonate
	Insulin and Glucose
	Kayexalate
	Diuretics (loop) and Dialysis
Hypercalcemia	IV hydration, loop diuretic ("loops lose calcium"), bisphosphonates (especially when caused by malignancy)
Hypokalemia	PO supplements, IV infusion of <10 mEq/h, K^+-sparing diuretics

| What electrolyte imbalance can result in hypokalemia refractory to supplementation? | Hypomagnesemia |
| Name the two classic PE findings associated with hypocalcemia. | Chvostek's sign (facial spasm upon tapping of facial nerve) and Trousseau's sign (carpal spasm upon arterial occlusion with BP cuff) |

Name the type of RTA associated with each of the following:

Decreased bicarbonate reabsorption	Type II (proximal)
Decreased H^+ excretion; nephrocalcinosis	Type I (distal)
Hyperkalemia	Type IV
Most common RTA	Type IV
Fanconi's syndrome	Type II (proximal)
Hyporeninemic hypoaldosteronism	Type IV
Seen commonly in diabetes mellitus	Type IV

Renal Failure

What are the three etiologies of ARF?	1. Prerenal (hypoperfusion)
	2. Intrinsic (renal)
	3. Postrenal (obstructive); can evaluate cause with renal U/S
Name five causes of prerenal ARF.	1. Hypovolemia
	2. Heart failure
	3. Sepsis
	4. Burns
	5. ↓ Renal blood flow (RBF) (e.g., ↓ CO, renal artery stenosis)

Name five causes of intrinsic ARF.	1. Acute tubular necrosis (ATN) 2. Acute interstitial nephritis 3. GN 4. Autoimmune vasculitis 5. Renal ischemia (e.g., thromboembolism)
Name three causes of postrenal ARF.	1. Prostate disease 2. Nephrolithiasis 3. Tumors
How is FE_{Na} calculated?	$(Urine_{Na+}/plasma_{Na+})/(urine_{Cr}/plasma_{Cr})$

Which type of ARF is associated with the following findings?

FE_{Na} <1%	Prerenal
FE_{Na} >4%	Postrenal
Hyaline urine casts	Prerenal
Muddy brown/granular casts	Intrinsic (ATN)
BUN:Cr ratio >20	Prerenal
Red cell casts	Intrinsic (GN)
White cell cast ± eosinophils	Intrinsic (allergic nephritis)
Enlarged prostate	Postrenal
⊕ ANCA	Intrinsic (vasculitis)
Urine osmolality >500	Prerenal

Name three types of insults to the proximal tubules that result in ATN.	1. Ischemia 2. Direct toxins (contrast dye, ampho B, aminoglycosides) 3. Myoglobinuria
What two classes of drugs most commonly cause interstitial nephritis?	Penicillins and nonsteroidal anti-inflammatory drugs (NSAIDs)
What unique UA finding is associated with drug-induced interstitial nephritis?	Eosinophilia
What lab value is used to diagnose and follow renal failure?	Creatinine

List the effects of uremia on the following systems:

Nervous system	Asterixis, confusion, seizures, coma
Cardiovascular system	Fibrinous pericarditis

Hematologic system	Anemia, immunosupression coagulopathy
GI system	Nausea, vomiting, gastritis
Dermatologic system	Pruritis, uremic frost (urea crystals on skin) in severe uremia
Endocrine system	Glucose intolerance
List six nonuremic complications of ARF.	1. Metabolic acidosis 2. Hyperkalemia → arrhythmias 3. Na^+ and H_2O excess → pulmonary edema and CHF 4. Hypocalcemia → osteodystrophy (from failure to secrete active vitamin D) 5. Anemia ($\downarrow$ erythropoietin [EPO] secretion) 6. HTN (from renin hypersecretion)
What are the indications for dialysis treatment?	**"AEIOUY"** Acidosis (unresponsive) Electrolyte abnormality (hyperkalemia) Ingestion of toxins Overload (fluid) Uremic symptoms (pericarditis, encephalopathy) Y-not?

Infections

What type of infection presents with flank pain, costovertebral angle tenderness, fever, dysuria, pyuria, bacteriuria?	Acute pyelonephritis
What are the two major causes of pylonephritis?	Ascending infection and hematogenous seeding
What are the most common organisms responsible for acute pyelonephritis?	*E. coli* > *Proteus* > *Enterobacter* (same as UTIs)
What is the greatest risk factor for pyelonephritis?	Vesicoureteric reflux (or incompetency)
List three possible sequelae of acute pyelonephritis.	1. Abscess 2. Renal papillary necrosis 3. Renal scars

What condition is characterized by broad renal scarring, loss of renal parenchyma over time, and thyroidization of kidneys?

Chronic pyelonephritis

Which renal disease presents with multiple 3–4-cm cysts in bilaterally enlarged kidneys resulting in chronic renal failure in adults?

Autosomal-dominant (adult) polycystic kidney disease (ADPKD); 50% have end-stage renal disease (ESRD) by age 60

What are the two most common presenting symptoms of ADPKD?

Pain and hematuria

What may the abdominal examination reveal in ADPKD?

Large palpable kidney

Name four other findings associated with ADPKD.

1. Cerebrovascular aneurysm
2. HTN
3. Nephrolithiasis
4. Mitral valve prolapse

What is the prognosis for autosomal-recessive polycystic kidney disease (PKD)?

Death in the first few years of life

Glomerular Disease

What syndrome is characterized by **hematuria**, ARF, HTN, and mild proteinuria?

Nephritic syndrome

What syndrome is characterized by **massive proteinuria** (>3.5 g/day), generalized edema, hyperlipidemia, and hypoalbuminemia?

Nephrotic syndrome

Classify each of the following statements as characteristics of nephrotic or nephritic syndrome:

Increased risk of infections

Nephrotic

Gross hematuria, oliguria

Nephritic

Anticoagulation therapy is indicated to reduce risk of DVT and renal vein thrombosis

Nephrotic

"Foamy urine"

Nephrotic

Transient oliguria usually followed by spontaneous diuresis

Nephritic

Hyperlipidemia, lipiduria

Nephrotic

Dyspnea and ascites

Nephrotic (severe edema)

One-third of cases associated with systemic diseases (lupus, diabetes, or amyloidosis)

Nephrotic

Smoky brown urine with RBC casts

Nephritic

Name the glomerulopathy most closely associated with the following findings:

GN with lens dislocation, nerve deafness, and posterior cataracts

Alport syndrome

Nodular glomerulosclerosis, glomerular capillary basement membrane thickening

Diabetic glomerulosclerosis (Kimmelstiel-Wilson disease)

Young African American males

Focal-segmental glomerulonephritis (FSGN)

C-ANCA

Wegener's granulomatosis

Most common cause of nephrotic syndrome in children

Minimal change disease (lipoid nephrosis)

Most common cause of ESRD in the United States

Diabetic glomerulosclerosis

Commonly associated with HIV infection, heroin addiction, sickle cell disease, and obesity

FSGN

Mesangial widening and recurrent hematuria and proteinuria

IgA nephropathy (Berger disease)

Associated with hepatitis C

Membranoproliferative glomerulonephritis (MPGN)

Responds well to steroids

Minimal change disease (aka steroid responsive nephropathy)

Responds to plasma exchange and pulsed steroids

Goodpasture's syndrome

X-linked recessive defect in α_5 chain of collagen type IV (COLA4A5)

Alport syndrome

Asymptomatic familial hematuria

Thin membrane disease GBM is only 50–60% of normal thickness)

"Wire loop lesions"

SLE—Lupus nephropathy, diffuse proliferative pattern

Upper-respiratory necrotizing vasculitis and granulomas

Wegener's granulomatosis

Increased ASO titer

Postinfectious GN

Most common glomerulopathy worldwide	IgA nephropathy (Berger disease)
Pulmonary hemorrhage and hemosiderin-filled macrophages in sputum	Goodpasture's syndrome
Associated with URI or GI infections, ↑ in kids	IgA nephropathy (Berger disease)
Associated with hepatitis B infection	Membranous GN
Antiglomerular basement membrane antibodies	Goodpasture's syndrome
Antinuclear antibody (ANA) ⊕	SLE
Immunofluorescence → granular IgG or C3 deposits	Postinfectious GN
Immunofluorescence → smooth, linear IgG deposits	Goodpasture's disease (crescentic GN)
Immunofluorescence → "spike and dome"	Membranous GN
GN associated with ↓ complement levels (3)	SLE, MPGN, postinfectious GN

Give the treatment for each of the following glomerulopathies:

FSGN	Supportive (protein and salt restriction, diuretic therapy, antihyperlipidemics) and prednisone
Postinfectious GN	Supportive (prognosis very good)
Wegener's granulomatosis	High-dose steroids and cytotoxic agents
IgA nephropathy	Steroids for flares (20% progress to ESRD)
SLE	Steroids, cyclophosphamide (for advanced types)

Renal Calculi

Name the type of renal calculus associated with each of the following findings:

1° hyperparathyroidism	Calcium phosphate
Idiopathic hypercalciuria	Calcium oxalate
Radiolucent stones	Uric acid

Staghorn calculi	Cysteine
Associated with *Proteus, Pseudomonas, Providencia,* and *Klebsiella* UTIs	Struvite $(Mg-NH_4-PO_4)$
Forms in acidic urine (pH <5.5)	Uric acid
Amino acid transport defect	Cysteine
Goat, myeloproliferative disease, or **chemotherapy**	Uric acid
Crohn's disease	Calcium oxalate
Xanthine oxidase deficiency	Uric acid

Name eight risk factors for nephrolithiasis.	1. ↓ fluid intake 2. Hypercalcemia 3. Gout 4. Enzyme deficiency 5. RTA 6. Medications (allopurinol, chemotherapy, loop diuretics) 7. Inflammatory bowel disease 8. ⊕ FH
What is the typical presentation of nephrolithiasis?	Acute onset, **severe**, colicky flank pain radiating to the groin with N/V and hematuria
Name three tests to evaluate for nephrolithiasis.	1. UA (hematuria, pH, crystals under microscope) 2. Abnormal XR (90% of stones are radiopaque) 3. Helical CT scan without contrast (now the **test of choice**)
What is the initial treatment for calculi?	**Hydration** and **analgesia**
What antihypertensive ↓ $[Ca^{2+}]$ in urine?	Thiazide diuretic
Stones up to what size can pass spontaneously?	Typically <5 mm
What is the treatment for stones >5 mm but <3 cm?	Extracorporeal shock wave lithotripsy (ESWL)

Urinary Tract

What is the most common malignant tumor of the urinary tract?	Bladder (transitional cell) cancer (↑ in males >60 y/o)
What is the strongest risk factor for urinary tract malignancies?	**Smoking** (also chronic infections, aniline dye, calculi)

What is the most common presenting symptom of bladder cancer?	Painless, gross hematuria
What is the diagnostic test of choice?	Cystoscopy
What is the etiology of squamous cell bladder cancers? (rare)	*Schistosoma haematobium*
Name four treatment options for bladder cancer.	1. Intravesical chemotherapy 2. Transurethral resection 3. Surgery ± radiation 4. Chemotherapy alone

Prostate

What is the most common cause of cancer in men?	Prostate cancer (lung > prostate in leading causes of cancer **death** in men)
What digital rectal examination (DRE) finding suggests prostate cancer?	Firm nodules
What is the histologic type of >95% of prostate cancers?	Adenocarcinoma
What percentage of patients with prostate cancer present with metastatic disease?	40% (most are initially asymptomatic)
What is the most common site of metastasis for prostate cancer?	Bone (vertebrae); must rule out in any elderly male with back pain
Why do obstructive symptoms occur less frequently than in BPH?	Cancer usually begins in the peripheral zone as opposed to BPH which occurs centrally
What serum marker is used to detect and follow prostate cancer?	Prostate specific antigen (PSA)
How is prostate cancer definitively diagnosed?	Transrectal biopsy of suspicious lesions
Name an alternative to prostatectomy for treatment of localized prostate cancer.	Radiation therapy
Name the two most common complications of prostatectomy.	Impotence and incontinence
List three treatment options for metastatic disease?	Androgen ablation: 1. Luteinizing hormone-releasing hormone (LHRH) agonists (leuprolide) 2. Antiantrogens (flutamide) 3. Orchiectomy
What are the screening recommendations for prostate cancer?	DRE and PSA every year >50 y/o (or >40 y/o if African American or ⊕ FH)

What are the two types of symptoms that result from BPH?	**Obstructive** (hesitancy, weak stream, incomplete emptying, urinary retention) and **irritative** (nocturia, ↑ frequency, urge incontinence, opening hematuria)
What may be found on PE in a patient with BPH?	Diffusely enlarged prostate
Is PSA helpful in monitoring BPH?	No (useful in posttreatment cancer patients)
Name four complications of BPH?	1. Bladder outlet obstruction 2. Urinary stasis (leading to infections and calculi) 3. Chronic urinary retention and overflow 4. Renal failure
What lab value can help detect obstructive uropathy?	Creatinine level (elevated if obstructive lesion)
What medical options are used to treat BPH?	5-α-Reductase inhibitors (finasteride) and α-receptor blockers (terazosin)
What are the indications for surgery in BPH?	Symptomatic obstruction: 1. Postvoid residual volume >100 mL 2. Multiple bouts of gross hematuria 3 Recurrent UTIs
Name the most common surgical procedure for BPH.	Transurethral resection of the prostate (TURP)

Erectile Dysfunction (ED)

Name the two categories of causes of ED.	**Primary** = never been able to have sustained erections; **Secondary** = acquired
Name three causes of primary ED.	1. Psychologic 2. Gonadal (↓ testosterone) 3. Endocrine (thyroid, Cushing, and so on)
Name three causes of 2° ED.	1. Drug-induced TCAs, diuretics, antipsychotics) 2. Vascular disease 3. Neurologic disease
Provide four treatment options for ED.	Sildenafil (or similar class), intracavernosal prostaglandins, vacuum-constriction device, or penile prosthesis

What drugs are an absolute contraindication for patients taking sildenafil?	Nitrates (co[...] lowering BF[...]

Testes

Name the testicular disorder associated with the following statements:

Failure of descent of testicle before 1 y/o; ↑ risk of cancer	Cryptorchidism
Malignant testicular tumor that is highly radiosensitive	**Sem**inomas = **Sen**sitive to radiation
Worst prognosis of all testicular tumors; highly invasive; elevated βHCG levels	Choriocarcinoma
Slow growing tumor usually discovered and removed before metastasis	Seminomas
Associated with an abnormally high attachment of the tunical vaginalis around the distal end of the spermatic cord (*bell clapper deformity*)	Testicular torsion (usually bilateral)
Usually presents as firm, painless mass	All testicular tumors
Rapid onset of testicular pain, swelling, and absence of flow on Doppler ultrasound	Testicular torsion (testicle unsalvageable after 6 h)
Bag of worms on testicular examination	Varicocele

Make the Diagnosis

25 y/o Asian male presents with N/V, and colicky right flank pain; PE: acute distress and costovertebral angle (CVA) tenderness; W/U: hematuria and discrete radiopacities on abdominal XR	Renal stones
45 y/o with documented h/o aortic atheromatous plaques presents with recent onset, severe left flank pain, and hematuria; Abdominal CT: wedge-shaped lesion in the left kidney	Renal infarct

...th long h/o DM presents ...creasing fatigue and edema; ↑ BP, retinopathy, and pitting edema; W/U: severe proteinuria and glycosuria	Diabetic nephropathy (glomerulosclerosis)
21 y/o sexually active female present with frequency and dysuria; PE: suprapubic tenderness; W/U: *E. coli* ⊕ urine cultures	UTI
25 y/o male presents with hemoptysis, dark urine, and fatigue; PE: bilateral crackles at lung bases; W/U: oliguria, hematuria, and anti-GBM Abs	Goodpasture's syndrome
7 y/o presents in stupor after ingesting antifreeze; PE: Kussmaul respirations and mental status changes; W/U reveals anion gap of 21 mEq/L	Metabolic acidosis (ethylene glycol toxicity)
6 y/o boy presents with hematuria and worsening vision; PE: corneal abnormalities, retinopathy, sensorineural hearing loss; W/U: hematuria with dysmorphic red cells	Alport syndrome
3 y/o boy with h/o recent URI presents with facial edema; PE: ascitic fluid in abdomen and pedal edema; W/U reveals 4+ proteinuria and ↓ serum albumin	Minimal change disease
70 y/o male recently started on an ACE inhibitor presents with weakness, N/V, and palpitations; PE: areflexia; ECG: tall peaked T waves and wide QRS complex	Hyperkalemia
65 y/o patient with h/o small cell lung cancer presents with lethargy, confusion, and seizures; W/U: Serum Na^+: <135 mEq/L, urinary Na^+ >20 meq/L, and urine osmolality >100 mOsm/kg	SIADH (hyponatremia)
A patient s/p parathyroidectomy presents with muscle cramps, dyspnea, and tetanic contraction; PE: facial spasm with tapping over facial nerve, carpal spasm with arterial occlusion by BP cuff; ECG: ↑ QT interval	Hypocalcemia
A patient on a loop diuretic for CHF presents with muscle weakness and cramps, fatigue, and ileus; PE: hyporeflexia, bradycardia; ECG: T-wave flattening, ST depression, and U waves	Hypokalemia

A patient hospitalized for CHF is started on an aminoglycoside for a UTI develops oliguria, N/V, and malaise; PE: $\uparrow$ BP and asterixis; serum electrolytes: $\uparrow$ Cr, K^+; UA: "muddy brown" casts, $FE_{Na}^+ >3\%$	ARF (drug-induced ATN)
70 y/o Black male with h/o of lifelong DM presents with peripheral edema, SOB, and oliguria; PE: auscultatory rales, pitting edema, myoclonus, and uremic frost; Serum electrolytes: $\uparrow$ Cr, hyperkalemia, hypocalcemia, hyperphosphatemia	Chronic renal failure
A female presents with fever, chills, and flank pain; PE: CVA tenderness; UA: leukocyte esterase $\oplus$, 30 WBC/hpf	Pyelonephritis
32 y/o male presents with pain and hematuria; PE: $\uparrow$ BP, palpable kidney, and midsystolic ejection click; Abdominal U/S: multiple cysts of renal parenchyma; cerebral angiogram: unruptured berry aneurysm	Polycystic kidney disease
12 y/o male with recent h/o sore throat presents with low urine output and dark urine; PE: periorbital edema; W/U: hematuria, $\uparrow$ BUN and Cr, $\uparrow$ ASO titer	Poststreptococcal GN
45 y/o Asian male with h/o hepatitis B presents with malaise, edema, and foamy urine; PE: anasarca; W/U proteinuria (>3.5 g/day), hyperlipiduria; hyperlipidemia, and hypoalbuminemia	Membranous GN
80 y/o male presents with urinary hesitancy, nocturia, and weak urinary stream; PE: diffusely enlarged rubbery prostate; Serum electrolytes: $\uparrow$ Cr; UA is within normal limits (WNL)	Benign Prostatic Hyperplasia (BPH)
68 y/o male smoker presents with flank pain and hematuria; PE: fever, palpable kidney mass; W/U: hypercalcemia, polycythemia	Renal cell carcinoma
20 y/o male presents with acute onset of left testicular pain and N/V; PE: swollen, tender testicular in transverse position, absent cremasteric reflex on L side; Doppler: no flow detected in L testicle	Testicular torsion

85 y/o male presents with back pain, weight loss, and weak urinary stream; PE: palpable firm nodule on DRE; W/U: ↑ PSA	Prostate cancer

ENDOCRINE

Pituitary

Name the pituitary disorder associated with each of the following:

Most common functional pituitary adenoma	Prolactinoma (adenoma)
Deficiency of gonadotropin-releasing hormone (GnRH) → no 2° sexual characteristics; associated with anosmia	Kallmann's syndrome
Polyuria, polydipsia, hypernatremia; associated with tumor, infection, and autoimmune disease	Central/neurogenic DI
Hypopituitarism from postpartum pituitary necrosis	Sheehan's syndrome
Enlargement of jaw, hands, feet, and coarsening facial features, with ↑ serum growth hormones (GH)	Acromegaly
Pituitary hypersecretion of ADH → hyponatremia, ↓ urine output, mental status changes	SIADH
What are the two general ways pituitary masses can present clinically?	1. Mass effects (bitemporal hemianopia, CN palsies) 2. Endocrine effects (e.g., amenorrhea, galactorrhea, hyperthyroidism, ↓ libido)
What is the treatment of choice for symptomatic nonprolactin secreting tumors?	Transspheniodal surgical resection
What is the medical treatment of choice for a prolactinoma?	Bromocriptine
What two proteins are used to diagnose acromegaly?	GH and IGF-1 (made in liver in response to GH)
What medical treatment is used to treat acromegaly?	Somatostatin (GH inhibitor)—used if no surgical cure

Patients with acromegaly are at increased risk for what type of malignancy?	Colonic polyps (close screening with colonoscopy is indicated)
What is the relationship between urine osmolality and serum osmolality in DI?	Low urine osmolality with high serum osmolality
How are psychogenic polydipsia and DI differentiated using a water deprivation test?	DI patients continue to produce a high volume of dilute urine while psychogenic polydipsia patients will no longer produce urine
What is the radiologic test of choice to detect pituitary abnormalities?	MRI (better soft-tissue resolution)
Which hormone level remains normal in panhypopituitarism?	Prolactin (under chronic inhibition by dopamine secreted by the hypothalamus)
Which hormones need to be replaced in panhypopituitarism?	Cortisol, levothyroxine, and estrogen or testosterone
Name five etiologies of SIADH.	1. CNS (head trauma, tumor, hydrocephalus) 2. Pulmonary (small cell lung CA, sarcoidosis, pneumonia, abscess) 3. Endocrine (Conn's syndrome, hypothyroidism) 4. Drugs (antipsychotics, antidepressants, oral hypoglycemics) 5. Surgery (intracranial, intrathoracic)
How is the diagnosis of SIADH made?	Urine osmolality >50–100 mOsm/kg (hyperosmolar urine), hyponatremia, and urinary sodium >20 mEq/L
What is the treatment for SIADH?	Fluid restriction and hypertonic saline (acutely); demeclocycline (chronic)
What is the treatment of DI?	DDAVP (desmopressin-an ADH analog), salt restriction, and ↑ water intake

Thyroid

Name four lab findings in hyperthyroidism.	↓ thyroid-stimulating hormone (TSH) (in 1°), ↑ free T4, ↑ total T4, ↑ T3 uptake
Name four lab findings in hypOthyroidism.	↑ TSH (very sensitive for 1°), ↓ free T4, ↓ total T4, ↓ T3 uptake

Describe how each of the following organ systems are affected by (1) Hypothyroidism (HypO) and (2) Hyperthyroidism:

Metabolism

HypO: Hypometabolic state, cold intolerance

Hyper: ↑ basal metabolic rate (BMR), heat intolerance

Cardiac

HypO: Exercise intolerance, ↓ HR, shortness of breath, pericardial effusion

Hyper: ↑ CO, ↑ HR, palpitations, cardiomegaly (long term)

Ocular

HypO: Periorbital myxedema

Hyper: Staring gaze, lid lag

Neuromuscular

HypO: hypoactive deep tendon reflexes (DTR)

Hyper: ↑ sympathetic activity, fine tremor

Skin

HypO: Coarse, dry skin; hair loss

Hyper: Warm, moist, and flushed skin; fine hair; Graves → pretibial myxedema

GI

HypO: Weight gain, constipation

Hyper: Weight loss despite hyperphagia, ↑ motility

Other

HypO: Menorrhagia, ↓ pitch of voice, depression

Hyper: Menstrual abnormalities, osteoporosis, anxiety

Name three possible treatments for hyperthyroidism.

1. Propranolol (control symptoms) followed by radioablation
2. Antithyroid drugs (methimazole, propylthrouvnel [PTU])
3. Thyroidectomy

What is the most common long-term side effect of radioablation or thyroidectomy?

HypOthyroidism

What is the treatment of choice for hypOthyroidism?

Levothyroxine

What feared complication of hyperthyroidism can be induced by an infection or surgery?

Thyroid storm (tachycardia, **high-output cardiac failure**, and coma)

What is the mortality rate of thyroid storm?	25%
What is the treatment of thyroid storm?	1. β-blockers 2. PTU 3. Iodine 4. Steroids

Name the thyroid disorder associated with each of the following statements:

Child with coarse facial features, short stature, mental retardation, and umbilical hernia	Congenital hypothyroidism (cretinism)
Goiter occurring with high frequency in iodine-deficient areas	Endemic goiter
Painless enlargement of thyroid of autoimmune etiology; requires long-term treatment with levothyroxine	Hashimoto's thyroiditis
Triad of diffuse thyroid hyperplasia, ophthalmopathy, dermopathy	Graves' disease
Postviral, painful inflammation of thyroid; usually self-limited, treated with ASA or corticosteroids	Subacute (granulomatous, de Quervain) thyroiditis
Painless goiter that can occur postpartum; can cause hypothyroidism	Subacute lymphocytic (painless) thyroiditis
Thyroid-stimulating immunoglobulin (TSI) and TSH-receptor AB	Graves' disease
Extreme thyroid enlargement (>2 kg) causing mass effects; most patients are euthyroid; may require surgical debulking	Multinodular goiter
Antimicrosomal AB, antithyroglobulin AB	Hashimoto's thyroiditis
Most common thyroid carcinoma	Papillary carcinoma
Calcitonin-secreting tumor in multiple endocrine neoplasia (MEN) syndromes	Medullary carcinoma
Carcinoma presenting as a single nodule with uniform follicles	Follicular carcinoma
Aggressive carcinoma of older patients with pleomophic cells; dismal prognosis	Anaplastic (undifferentiated) carcinoma

Which two types of thyroid cancer have the worst prognosis?	Medullary and anaplastic
What is the test of choice for the detection of metastases from thyroid malignancies?	Radioactive iodine scan
What is the treatment for a malignant thyroid nodule?	Surgical resection
Are most thyroid nodules benign or malignant?	Benign
What findings are associated with ↑ risk of thyroid cancer?	1. Prior neck radiation 2. **Cold** nodule 3. Firm, fixed, rapidly growing solitary nodule 4. Hoarseness/dysphagia
What is the diagnostic test of choice to evaluate a thyroid nodule?	Fine needle aspiration (FNA)

Name the MEN syndrome described below:

Pheochromocytoma, thyroid medullary carcinoma, and parathyroid adenomas	MEN 2 (Sipple's syndrome)
Tumors of the pituitary, pancreatic islet cells, and parathyroids	MEN 1 (Wermer's syndrome)
Tumors in MEN2 plus tall, thin habitus, prominent lips, and ganglioneuromas of the tongue and eyelids	MEN 3 (MEN 2b)
AD inheritance	All MEN syndromes

Parathyroid

Name the parathyroid disorder associated with each of the following statements:

Caused by chronic renal failure or ↓ vitamin D	$2°$ hyperparathyroidism
Most commonly due to parathyroid adenomas (90%)	$1°$ hyperparathyroidism
Etiologies include congenital gland absence, postsurgical, and autoimmune destruction	HypOparathyroidism
Caused by an autonomous hormone secreting adenoma	$3°$ hyperparathyroidism

Autosomal recessive (AR) end-organ resistance to PTH → short stature and short third/fourth metacarpals	Pseudohypoparathyroidism
What four systems are primarily affected by hyperparathyroidism?	"Painful bones, renal stones, abdominal groans, and psychic moans" **Painful bones:** Osteitis fibrosa cystica, osteoporosis **Renal stones:** Nephrolithiasis, nephrocalcinosis **Abdominal groans:** Constipation, peptic ulcer disease (PUD), pancreatitis **Psychic moans:** Depression, lethargy, seizures
What is the treatment of chronic symptomatic hypercalcemia from hyperparathyroidism?	Parathyroidectomy with preoperative bisphosphonates
Name two postoperative complications of parathyroidectomy.	Recurrent laryngeal nerve injury (hoarseness) and hypOcalcemia

Adrenals and Steroids

Name the four etiologies for hypercortisolism.	1. Exogenous glucocorticoids (most common overall) 2. Pituitary ACTH hypersecretion (e.g., adenoma) 3. Hypersecretion of cortisol (e.g., adrenal hyperplasia) 4. Ectopic ACTH (e.g., small cell lung cancer)
What is the most common cause of endogenous hypercortisolism?	Cushing's **disease** ($1°$ pituitary adenoma)
Name eight classic clinical findings of Cushing's syndrome.	1. Hyperglycemia/hypokalemia/HTN 2. Virilization and menstrual disorder in women 3. Moon facies 4. Truncal obesity 5. Buffalo hump 6. Skin changes (thinning, striae) 7. Osteoporosis—vertebral compression fractures 8. Immune suppression-susceptibility to infection

What two tests are used to screen for Cushing's syndrome?

Overnight low-dose dexamethasone suppression test and 24-h urine-free cortisol

What test is used to localize the source of hypercortisolism?

1. Check ACTH levels ($\uparrow$ = ectopic/pituitary; $\downarrow$ = adrenal)
2. High-dose dexamethasone suppression test (when ACTH $\uparrow$, suppression suggests pituitary disease)

Name the adrenal disorder associated with each of the following statements:

Aldosterone-secreting adenoma causing HTN, hypokalemic, hypernatremia, and metabolic alkalosis

Conn's syndrome ($1°$ hyperaldosteronism)

Endotoxin-mediated massive adrenal hemorrhage

Waterhouse-Friderichsen syndrome (caused by *Neisseria meningitidis*)

Deficiency of aldosterone and cortisol occurs $2°$ to adrenal atrophy or autoimmune destruction; may cause hypotension

$1°$ chronic adrenocortical insufficiency (Addison's disease)

Hypothalamic-pituitary axis (HPA) disturbance causing failure of ACTH secretion

$2°$ adrenocortical insufficiency

Bilateral hyperplasia of zona glomerulosa caused by stimulation of RAA system

$2°$ hyperaldosteronism

Results from rapid steroid withdrawal or sudden $\uparrow$ in glucocorticoid requirements

$1°$ acute adrenocortical insufficiency (adrenal crisis)

Chromaffin cell tumor usually in adults; results in episodic hyperadrenergic symptoms

Pheochromocytoma

Malignant, small, round, blue cell tumor of medulla in kids associated with N-*myc* oncogene amplification

Neuroblastoma

How is $1°$ and $2°$ adrenocortical insufficiency differentiated?

$2°$ is not associated with hyperpigmentation

What substance can be measured to differentiate between $1°$ and $2°$ hyperaldosteronism?

Renin ($\uparrow$ in $2°$ hyperaldosteronism)

What is the drug of choice for hyperaldosteronism?	Spironolactone (aldosterone antagonist)
What is the "rule of 10s" for pheochromocytomas?	10% malignant
	10% bilateral
	10% extraadrenal
	10% kids
	10% familial
	10% calcify
What are the five Ps of pheochromocytoma (symptoms)?	Pressure, Pain (headache), Perspiration, Palpitations, and Pallor
What substances are secreted from pheochromocytomas and how are they detected?	Epinephrine and norepinephrine; diagnosed by ↑ urinary secretion of catecholamines and their metabolites (metanephrine, VMA, and so on)
What is the treatment of a pheochromocytoma?	Surgical resection (preoperative α and β-blockade)
Why is it necessary to block α-receptors before giving a β-blocker?	To prevent unopposed vasoconstriction
What are the electrolyte and CBC abnormalities in Addison's disease?	Hyponatremia, hyperkalemia, and eosinophilia
What test is used to evaluate the etiology of Addison's disease?	ACTH stimulation test (↑ ACTH and ↓ cortisol = Addison's; ↓ ACTH and ↑ cortisol = $2°$ cause)
What is the treatment of adrenal insufficiency?	Replacement of glucocorticoids and mineral corticoids
What must be administered to a patient with Addison's disease during periods of stress (e.g., surgery, trauma, or infection)?	Stress-dose steroids
What are the two main etiologies of $1°$ hyperaldosteronism and their respective treatments?	Adrenal adenoma (Conn's syndrome) → adrenalectomy; bilateral hyperplasia → spironolactone

Pancreas-Diabetes Mellitus

What endocrine disease should be suspected in a patient who presents with poor wound healing or recurrent vaginal candidiasis?	Diabetes Mellitus (DM)
Describe the classic acute presentation of type 1 diabetes mellitus.	Polydipsia, polyuria, polyphagia, weight loss, and DKA if extreme

What is the proposed mechanism of islet cell destruction in type 1 DM?	Environmental triggering of autoimmunity to islet β-cells
What is the theorized cause of type 2 DM?	Obesity increases insulin resistance and causes β-cell dysfunction
Name three criteria to diagnose DM.	1. Fasting glucose >126 mg/dL 2. Random glucose >200 mg/dL with symptoms 3. 2-h glucose >200 mg/dL during 75 g oral glucose tolerance test (on two separate occasions)
What is HbA$_{1c}$ and what is it used for?	Percent of glycosylated hemoglobin in blood; used to measure diabetic control over last 90–120 days (average lifespan of RBC)—goal <8%

Name the acute complication of DM described below:

Abdominal pain, vomiting, Kussmaul respirations, fruity odor, anion gap metabolic acidosis, and mental status changes usually precipitated by stress (infection, drugs, MI, or noncompliance with insulin therapy)	DKA—type 1 DM
Profound dehydration, extreme hyperglycemia, mental status changes without acidosis	Hyperosmolar hyperglycemic nonketotic coma (HHNK)—type 2 DM
What are the three major components of the treatment of DKA?	Fluids (add dextrose when glucose falls below 200 mg/dL), insulin, and potassium
Why must K^+ be replaced in a patient with DKA even through serum levels are usually elevated?	Acidosis and insulonopenia force K^+ out of cells initially but the total body potassium levels may be low
What is the mortality rate of HHNK?	50%
What is the main treatment of HHNK?	Aggressive fluid replacement

Describe the effect of long-term DM on each of the following organ systems:

Cardiovascular (macrovascular)	Atherosclerosis → CVA, MI, PVD
Urinary (microvascular)	Glomerular (glomerulosclerosis, proteinuria); vascular (arteriosclerosis → HTN, CRF); infectious (UTIs, pyelonephritis, necrotizing papillitis)

Nervous (microvascular)	Motor and sensory peripheral neuropathy, autonomic degeneration/dysfunction (orthostatic hypotension)
Eye (microvascular)	Retinopathy, cataract formation, blindness
Skin	Xanthomas, abscesses from ↑ infections and poor wound healing, fungal infections

What two factors are shown to correlate with the severity of microvascular complications?

1. Glycemic control
2. Duration of disease

What preventive measures must be taken to minimize complications of DM?

1. Yearly fundoscopic examination
2. Periodic UA
3. Proper foot care
4. BP control (<135/85)
5. Lipid control (LDL <130, TGs <200)

Name the appropriate therapy for each of the following clinical scenarios in a diabetic:

Proliferative retinopathy	Laser photocoagulation
Microalbuminuria	ACE inhibitor or ARB
Neuropathy	Gabapentin and amitriptyline
Type 1 diabetes	Insulin
Newly diagnosed type 2 diabetes refractory to lifestyle modifications	Oral hypoglycemics
Type 2 diabetes refractory to monotherapy with an oral hypoglycemic agent	Oral hypoglycemic agent with a different mechanism or begin insulin therapy

For each of the following types of insulin, state the peak and duration of action:

Insulin lispro	Peak = 15–30 min; duration = 3–4 h
NPH insulin	Peak = 8–12 h; duration = 18–24 h
Lente insulin	Peak = 8–12 h; duration = 18–24 h
Ultralente insulin	Peak = 8–16 h; duration = 18–28 h
Insulin glargine	Peak = none (peakless); duration >24 h

For each oral hypoglycemic, state the mechanism and unique toxicity of each:

    Biguanides (e.g., metformin)

↓ hepatic gluconeogenesis and ↑ peripheral uptake of glucose; of risk lactic acidosis in pts with renal disease, hepatic disease and contrast dye

    Sulfonylureas (e.g., glyburide, glipizide, glimepiride)

↑ insulin secretion; may cause hypoglycemia

    Thiazolidinediones (e.g., pioglitazone, rosiglitazone)

↑ peripheral insulin responsiveness; may cause hepatotoxicity

    α-Glucosidase inhibitors (e.g., acarbose, miglitol)

↓ GI absorption of carbohydrates; may cause GI upset/flatulence

Name four causes of 2° diabetes mellitus.

1. Pancreatic disease (e.g., hemochromatosis, pancreatitis, pancreatic carcinoma)
2. Pregnancy (gestational diabetes)
3. Cushing's syndrome
4. Other endocrine disorders (e.g., acromegaly, glucagonoma, hyperthyroidism)

Name the following complications of diabetic management:

    Nocturnal hypoglycemia causing elevated morning glucose 2° to release of counterregulatory hormones

Somogyi effect

    Abrupt early-morning hyperglycemia caused by reduced effectiveness of insulin

Dawn phenomenon

Name the islet cell tumor associated with each of the following statements:

    Most common is let cell tumor

Insulinoma (β-cell tumor)

    2° diabetes mellitus, necrolytic migratory erythema

Glucagonoma (α-cell tumor)

    Associated with ZE syndrome

Gastrinoma

    Associated with WDHA (watery diarrhea, hypokalemia, and achlorhydria) syndrome

VIPoma

    2° diabetes mellitus, cholelithiasis, steatorrhea

Somatostatinoma (δ-cell tumor)

Clinically characterized by Whipple's triad

Insulinoma (β-cell tumor)

Name the clinical findings of Whipple's triad.

Hypoglycemia, concurrent CNS dysfunction, and reversal of CNS symptoms with glucose

What is ZE syndrome?

Hypersecretion of gastric HCl, recurrent PUD, and hypergastinemia (associated with MEN)

How is ZE syndrome diagnosed?

↑ serum gastin level with secretin stimulation test

Make the Diagnosis

31 y/o presents with loss of libido, galactorrhea, and irregular menses; PE: bitemporal hemianopia; W/U: negative βHCG

Prolactinoma

Patient presents to clinic with polyuria and polydipsia; W/U: urine specific gravity <1.005, urine osmolality <200 mOsm/kg, hypernatremia

Diabetes Insipidus (DI)

30 y/o White female presents with weight loss, tremor, and palpitations; PE: brisk DTR, ophthalmopathy, pretibial myxedema; W/U: ↓ TSH, ↑ T4, ↑ T3 index

Grave's disease

40 y/o female presents with fatigue, constipation, and weight loss; PE: puffy face, cold dry hands, coarse hair, and enlargement of thyroid gland; W/U: ↑ TSH, ↓ T3 and T4, ⊕ antimicrosomal AB and antithyroglobulin AB

Hashimoto's disease

32 y/o female with h/o recurrent PUD presents with episodes of hypocalcemia and nephrolithiasis; W/U: fasting hypoglycemia, ↑ gastrin levels, and hypercalcemia

MEN 1

70 y/o presents with episodal HTN, nephrolithiasis, and diarrhea; PE: ↑ BP, thyroid nodule; W/U: ↑ calcitonin levels, ↑ urinary catecholamines

MEN 2

A female patient presents with bone pain, kidney stones, depression, and recurrent ulcers; W/U: hypercalcemia, hypophosphatemia, and hypercalciuria	Hyperparathyroidism
35 y/o female presents with weight gain, irregular menses, and HTN; PE: $\uparrow$ BP, weight in face and upper back, hirsutism, multiple ecchymoses; W/U: $\uparrow$ ACTH levels and suppression with high-dose dexamethasone suppression test	Cushing's disease
45 y/o with recent h/o coarsening of facial features presents with headaches and states that his shoes no longer fit; PE: enlarged jaw, tongue, hands and feet, and bitemporal hemianopia	Acromegaly
9 y/o female presents with muscle cramps; PE: rounded face with flat nasal bridge, abnormal dentition, positive Trousseau's sign and Chvostek's sign, and shortened metacarpals	Albright hereditary osteodystrophy (pseudohypoparathyroidism)
50 y/o female presents with HTN, muscle weakness, and fatigue; W/U: hypokalemia, hypernatremia, and metabolic alkalosis	Conn's syndrome
30 y/o female presents with progressive weakness, weight loss, N/V; PE: hyperpigmentation of skin, $\downarrow$ BP; W/U: hyperkalemia, hyponatremia, and eosinophilia	Addison's disease
40 y/o presents with episodes of HA, diaphoresis, palpitations, and tremor; PE: $\uparrow$ BP, $\uparrow$ HR; W/U: $\uparrow$ in urinary VMA and homovanillic acid	Pheochromocytoma
17 y/o White female with h/o DM presents with diffuse abdominal pain, N/V, and slight confusion; PE: $\downarrow$ BP, shallow rapid breathing pattern; W/U: glucose = 300, hypokalemia, hypophosphatemia, and metabolic acidosis	DKA-DM type I

60 y/o diabetic obese patient found at home confused and disoriented; PE: ↓ BP, ↑ HR; W/U: glucose >1000, pH is WNL	HHNK-DM type II
50 y/o female presents with h/o weakness, blurred vision, and confusion several h after meals, which improves with eating; W/U: ↑ fasting levels of insulin and hypoglycemia	Insulinoma

HEMATOLOGY/ONCOLOGY

Anemias

What are some common presenting symptoms in an anemic patient?	Fatigue, DOE, angina, headache, dizziness, and syncope
List five of the most common causes of microcytic anemia.	Iron deficiency, lead poisoning, chronic disease (sometimes normocytic), sideroblastic, thalassemia
List four of the most common causes of normocytic anemia.	Sickle cell, aplastic, acute blood loss, hemolytic anemia
List five of the most common causes of macrocytic anemia.	Liver disease, vitamin B_{12} deficiency, folate deficiency, alcoholism, hypothyroidism
What is the primary site of iron absorption?	Duodenum
What are the two most common causes of iron deficiency anemia in adults?	Menorrhagia or GI blood loss
What is the mechanism of ischemic necrosis of the bones, lungs, liver, brain, spleen, or penis in sickle cell disease?	↓ O_2 tension → abnormal RBCs sickle → microvascular occlusions
What two common enzyme deficiencies can cause hemolytic anemia?	Glucose-6-phosphate dehydrogenase and pyruvate kinase deficiency
What two autoimmune conditions of the GI tract can cause megaloblastic anemia?	Pernicious anemia (due to lack of intrinsic factor [IF] production) and Crohn's disease (due to lack of IF-B_{12} complex reabsorption in distal ileum)
How does gastric resection cause megaloblastic anemia?	Parietal cells, which are responsible for IF production may be removed when the gastric fundus is resected

Name the type(s) of anemia associated with the following clinical or pathologic features:

Abnormal Schilling test	Pernicious anemia
Angular chelitis, koilonychia, pica	Iron deficiency anemia
Autosplenectomy	Sickle cell anemia
Basophilic stipling of erythrocytes, blue/gray discoloration at gumline, wrist/foot drop	Microcytic anemia (lead poisoning)
Celiac sprue	Megaloblastic (folate deficiency) and iron deficiency anemias
Chronic atrophic gastritis	Pernicious anemia
Colon cancer	Iron deficiency anemia (early) and anemia of chronic disease (late)
Crescent-shaped erythrocytes and Howell-Jolly bodies	Sickle cell anemia
↓ Serum iron, normal iron-binding protein saturation, ↓ ferritin, ↓ TIBC	Anemia of chronic disease
↓ Ferritin, ↑ RDW, ↑ TIBC, ↓ Serum iron, ↓ iron-binding protein saturation	Iron deficiency anemia
↑ Serum iron, maximal iron-binding protein saturation, ↑ ferritin, **normal TIBC**	Iron overload/hereditary hemochromatosis
Deficiency of α or β globin gene synthesis	Thalassemia
Deficiency of decay accelerating factor	Paroxysmal nocturnal hemoglobinuria
Demyelination of the dorsal and lateral tracts of the spinal cord	Pernicious anemia
Diphyllobothrium latum (fish tapeworm) and *G. lamblia* infection	Macrocytic anemia (B_{12} deficiency)
↑ reticulocyte count, indirect hyperbilirubinemia, ↑ LDH, and negative direct Coombs' test	Hemolytic anemia
End-stage liver disease	Macrocytic anemia
Oxidative stress on erythrocytes in a G6PD-deficient patient	Hemolytic anemia
"Fishmouth vertebrae" on radiograph	Sickle cell anemia

Gastric carcinoma	Pernicious anemia
Glossitis and peripheral neuropathy	Pernicious anemia
Helmet cells, burr cells, triangular cells	Microangiopathic anemia ($2°$ to disseminated intravascular coagulation [DIC], TTP-HUS), or mechanical heart valves)
Persistently elevated creatinine	Anemia of chronic renal failure
High reticulocyte count	Hemolytic anemia (or acute hemorrhage)
Hypersegmented PMNs	Vitamin B_{12} or folate deficiency anemia
Hypothyroidism	Macrocytic anemia
Leukemias and lymphomas	Autoimmune hemolytic anemia
Fatigue, jaundice, dark urine after consumption of fava beans	Hemolytic anemia (due to G6PD deficiency)
Pancytopenia and fatty infiltration of bone marrow	Aplastic anemia
Malaria or babesiosis	Hemolytic anemia
May be caused by Crohn's disease of the terminal ileum	Macrocytic anemia (B_{12} deficiency)
Microcytosis, atrophic glossitis, esophageal webs (Plummer-Vinson triad)	Iron deficiency anemia (long standing)
Most common type of anemia	Iron deficiency anemia
M. pneumoniae infection	Cold autoimmune hemolytic anemia
NSAIDs, chloramphenicol use	Aplastic anemia
Penicillin, cephalosporin, or quinidine use	Autoimmune hemolytic anemia
AD deficiency of spectrin, positive osmotic fragility test	Hereditary spherocytosis
Priapism	Sickle cell anemia
SLE, chronic lymphocytic leukemia (CLL), lymphomas, drugs; ⊕ direct Coombs' test (due to IgG autoantibodies)	Warm autoimmune hemolytic anemia
Reduced erythropoietin	Anemia of chronic disease
Ringed sideroblasts	Sideroblastic anemia
Schistocytes	Microhemangiopathic anemia

Susceptibility to infection by encapsulated organisms	Sickle cell anemia (due to functional asplenia)
Target cells	Liver disease, thalassemia, hemolysis
Unconjugated bilirubinemia, ↑ urine urobilinogen, ↓ hemoglobin, hemoglobinuria, ↓ haptoglobin, hemosiderosis	Hemolytic anemia

Name the type of thalassemia responsible for each of the following findings:

β-Thalassemia associated with growth retardation, frontal bossing and HSM (from extramedullary hematopoesis), jaundice, and iron overload ($2°$ to transfusions), and ↑ Hgb F	β-Thalassemia major (β-/β-); **Note:** β-Thalassemia minor (β+/β-) typically asymptomatic
α-Thalassemia associated with mild microcytic anemia, usually asymptomatic	α-Thalassemia minor (two alleles affected); **Note:** When only one allele involved (carrier state) → no anemia
α-Thalassemia associated with pallor, splenomegaly, chronic hemolytic anemia, and intraerythrocytic inclusions	Hgb H disease (three alleles affected)
α-Thalassemia associated with stillborn fetus	Hydrops fetalis (all four alleles affected)

Name three infectious and three noninfectious complications of sickle cell disease.

Infectious:

1. Osteomyelitis (usually due to *Salmonella*)
2. Pneumococcal and *H. influenzae* pneumonia
3. Parvovirus B_{19} infection causing aplastic anemia

Noninfectious:

1. High-output cardiac failure
2. Splenomegaly (in infants)
3. Vasoocclusive crises

What is the treatment of a vasoocclusive sickle crisis?	Oxygen therapy, IV hydration, analgesia (usually opioids)
What treatment may be used in the setting of severe vasoocclusive crises and chest syndrome with respiratory distress?	Exchange transfusions

What chemotherapeutic agent may decrease the frequency of sickle cell crises?	Hydroxyurea

Coagulation Disorders

Name the coagulation disorder associated with the following clinical features:

Classic triad of thrombocytopenia, hemolytic anemia, and ARF	Hemolytic-uremic syndrome (HUS)
Classic triad of HUS + fever and neurologic changes	TTP; **Remember: "FAT RN"** Fever, Anemia (hemolytic), Thrombocytopenia, Renal failure, Neurologic abnormalities
Commonly follows viral URI in children but may be chronic in adults	Idiopathic thrombocytopenic purpura (ITP)
Commonly occurs in the context of sepsis, major hemorrhage (traumatic or obstetric), or malignancies	DIC
X-linked disorder characterized by hemarthroses and GI bleeding; ↑ PTT, normal PT, platelet count, and bleeding time	Hemophilia
AD disorder characterized by episodes of easy bruising, mucosal and GI bleeding	von Willebrand's disease
Treated with Factor VIII	Hemophilia A
Treated with Factor IX	Hemophilia B
Commonly in children; may be caused by *E. coli* O157:H7	HUS
Spontaneous bleeding from surgical wounds and venipuncture sites	DIC
Associated with lymphomas, leukemias, HIV infection, and autoimmune diseases	ITP
IgG antiplatelet antibodies (⊕ Coombs)	ITP
↑ bleeding time, ↓ Factor VIII, normal platelet count, normal PT and PTT	von Willebrand's disease
Prolonged PT, PTT, ↑ fibrin split products (D-dimer), ↓ Hct, ↓ platelets	DIC (also known as "consumptive coagulopathy")

Schistocytes, ↑ unconjugated bilirubin, ↑ LDH	TTP
First-line therapy = oral steroids; second line is IV immunoglobulin (IVIG), splenectomy, or chemotherapy (commonly, cyclophosphamide)	ITP
First-line therapy = plasmapheresis or IVIG; splenectomy for refractory cases (fatal if untreated)	TTP
Treatment aimed at underlying disorder; treatment for coagulopathy with platelet transfusion, cryoprecipitate; Second line = aminocaproic acid	DIC
Mild disease treated with desmopressin; severe disease treated with Factor VIII concentrate	von Willebrand's disease

WBC Neoplasia

Name the general type of lymphoma (Hodgkin's or Non-Hodgkin's lymphoma [NHL]) associated with the following clinical and pathologic features:	
Reed Sternberg (RS) cells secreting interleukin (IL-5)	Hodgkin's disease (HD)
Peak incidence from 20 to 40 years of age, more common in women	NHL
Bimodal age distribution but most common in young men	HD
Constitutional symptoms including fever, night sweats, weight loss	Both
Mediastinal lymphadenopathy, contiguous spread	HD
Systemic adenopathy	NHL
Regional lymphadenopathy	HD
Associated with EBV, HIV infection	HD
Peripheral lymphadenopathy, noncontiguous spread	NHL

| Lymphadenopathy may become painful with alcohol consumption | HD |
| Associated with immunosuppression including AIDS | NHL |

Leukemias and Lymphomas

Name the general type of leukemia (acute or chronic) associated with the following clinical and pathologic features:	
Immature blast cells predominate	Acute
Mature cell types predominate	Chronic
Bimodal age distribution	Acute
Rapid onset and quickly progressive disease	Acute
Indolent course	Chronic
Common in middle adulthood	Chronic

What are the three most common medical complications of end-stage leukemia?	1. Hemorrhage (due to thrombocytopenia) 2. Infection (due to immunosupression) 3. Anemia (due to involvement of bone marrow)

Name the specific leukemia associated with each of the following demographics:	
Most common leukemia of childhood, peak age 3–4 y/o	Acute lymphocytic leukemia (ALL)
Most common leukemia in adults	Acute myelogenous leukemia (AML)
Commonly in males 60 and older	CLL

Name the specific leukemia associated with each of the following findings:	
Very high white cell counts, often >200,000	Chronic myelogenous leukemia (CML)
Isolated lymphocytosis	CLL
TdT positive lymphoblasts	ALL
Large, immature myeloblasts predominate	AML
Smudge cells	CLL

Bone marrow is replaced with myeloblasts	AML
Philadelphia chromosome t(9:22)	CML
Auer rods	AML
Low leukocytic alkaline phosphatase	CML (as well as paroxysmal nocturnal hematuria)
Associated with fatigue, thrombocytopenia (easy bruising), signs of anemia, frequent infections, leukemia cutis, and DIC	AML
Bone pain, fever, generalized lymphadenopathy, HSM and signs of CNS spread	ALL
Excellent prognosis if treated early	ALL
May progress to AML	CML
Most responsive to therapy	ALL
Associated with prior exposure to radiation	CML
Peripheral leukocytes containing tartarate resistant acid phosphatase and cytoplasmic projections	Hairy cell leukemia

Myeloproliferative Disorders

Name the four chronic myeloproliferative disorders.	1. Chronic myelogenous leukemia 2. Polycythemia vera 3. Essential thrombocytosis 4. Myelofibrosis with myeloid metaplasia
Name the myeloproliferative disorder associated with each of the following clinical and pathologic findings:	
↑ RBC mass and low/normal erythropoietin	Polycythemia vera
Tear drop deformity of erythrocytes, bone marrow hypercellularity	Myelofibrosis with myeloid metaplasia
Plethoric complexion, pruritus after showering, epistaxis, blurred vision, splenomegaly, and epistaxis	Polycythemia vera
Erythromelalgia (throbbing or burning of hands and feet)	Essential thrombocytosis

Basophilia	Polycythemia vera
Widespread extramedullary hematopoesis with megakaryocytic proliferation in the bone marrow	Myelofibrosis with myeloid metaplasia
Hyperviscosity syndrome	Polycythemia vera and essential thrombocytosis
Peripheral thrombocytosis, bone marrow megakaryocytosis, and splenomegaly	Essential thrombocytosis
Treated with ASA, phlebotomy, and/or hydroxyurea	Polycythemia vera
Treated with platelet exchange (for acute exacerbations), hydroxyurea, and anagrelide	Essential thrombocytosis

Name the plasma cell disorder associated with the following clinical and pathologic findings:

Bone pain, osteopenia, pathologic fractures, and "punched-out" lytic lesions on x-ray	Multiple myeloma
Russel bodies and "plymphocytes" (plasmacytoid lymphocytes)	Waldenstrom macroglobulinemia
Bence-Jones proteinuria	Multiple myeloma and Waldenstrom macroglobulinemia
Small M-spike on plasma electrophoresis in an otherwise healthy patient	Monoclonal gammopathy of undetermined significance (MGUS)
Hypercalcemia; renal insufficiency	Multiple myeloma
Hyperviscosity syndrome	Waldenstrom macroglobulinemia
Large M-spike on plasma electrophoresis	Multiple myeloma and Waldenstrom macroglobulinemia
Primary amyloidosis	Multiple myeloma

Name the disease or condition associated with each of the following peripheral blood smear findings:

Atypical lymphocytes	Infectious mononucleosis
Auer rods	AML (M3 subtype)
Basophilic stippling	Lead poisoning
Burr cells (echinocytes)	Burns, uremia

Heinz bodies	G6PD deficiency
Helmet cells, schistocytes	Microangiopathic hemolytic anemia (DIC, TTP, HUS)
Howell-Jolly bodies	Pernicious anemia
Hypersegmented PMN nuclei	Megaloblastic anemia
Lymphocytic cerebriform nuclei	Sézary syndrome
Nucleated erythrocytes	Hemolytic anemia
Rouleau formation	Multiple myeloma and Waldenstrom macroglobulinemia
Smudge cells	CLL
Spherocytes	Hereditary spherocytosis and hemolytic anemia
Spur cells (acanthocytes)	Abetalipoproteinemia, liver disease
Target cells (codocytes)	Thalassemias, iron deficiency anemia, liver disease, sickle cell anemia
Teardrop cells (dacrocytes)	Myelofibrosis
Toxic granulations in leukocytes	Severe infection

Make the Diagnosis

50 y/o with h/o bone marrow transplant for CML 3 weeks ago presents with severe pruritis, diarrhea, and jaundice; PE: violaceous rash on palms and soles; W/U: ↑ bilirubin, ALT, and AST	Graft-versus-host disease
1 y/o Greek child presents with pallor and delayed milestones; PE: pallor, skeletal abnormalities, splenomegaly; peripheral blood smear (PBS): hypochromic microcytic RBCs; target cells, fragmented RBCs; Skull XR: "hair-on-end" appearance	β-Thalassemia
10 y/o with a h/o recurrent chest pain presents with fever and bilateral leg pain; PE: febrile, multiple leg ulcers; PBS shows sickle shaped erythrocytes; Hb electrophoresis shows HbS band	Sickle cell anemia

60 y/o with headache, vertigo, blurry vision, pruritus, joint pain; PE: ↑ BP, plethoric, splenomegaly; W/U: Hct = 60, mild leukocytosis, and hyperuricemia

Polycythemia vera

4 y/o male with a 1 week h/o fever, pallor, headache, and bone tenderness; PE: fever, HSM, and generalized nontender lymphadenopathy; W/U; PBS reveals absolute lymphocytosis with abundant TdT ⊕ lymphoblasts

Acute lymphoblastic leukemia

27 y/o presents with 2-month h/o fatigue, oropharyngeal candidiasis, pseudomonal UTI, and epistaxis; PE: numerous petechiae and ecchymoses of skin, gingival mucosal bleeding, guaiac ⊕ stools; W/U: ↑ WBCs, PBS shows >30% myeloblasts with Auer rods

Acute myelocytic leukemia

17 y/o male presents with a 2-month h/o fever, night sweats, and weight loss; PE: nontender, cervical lymphadenopathy, and HSM; CBC: leukocytosis; CXR: bilateral hilar adenopathy; Lymph node biopsy: Reed-Sternberg cells

Hodgkin's disease

60 y/o male presents with fatigue and anorexia; PE: generalized lymphadenopathy and HSM; CBC: WBC: 250,000, ⊕ direct Coombs' test; PBS: small, round lymphocytes predominate with occasional smudge cells

Chronic lymphocytic leukemia

10 y/o Black child presents with a 3-week h/o a rapidly enlarging, painless mandibular mass; CBC: mild anemia and leukopenia; Cytogenetics reveal a t(8:14) translocation; Excisional biopsy: "starry-sky" pattern

Burkitt's lymphoma

35 y/o presents with a 3-year h/o mild weight loss, anorexia presents with worsening DOE; PE: splenomegaly; CBC: mild anemia, WBC = 125,000; PBS: granulocytosis with <10% myeloblasts; Cytogenetics reveal a t(9:22) translocation

Chronic myelocytic leukemia

55 y/o with a recent h/o streptococcal pneumonia presents with bone pain and weight loss; W/U: mild anemia, hypercalcemia; PBS: roleau formation; UA: Bence-Jones proteinuria; serum electrophoresis: M-spike; XR: cranial "punched-out" lesions

Multiple myeloma

18 y/o female develops dyspnea and declining mental status 1 h after a C-section complicated by excess blood loss; PE: mucosal bleeding, large clot in the vaginal vault; coags: ↑ PT and PTT, ↓ platelets, ↑ fibrin split products

Disseminated intravascular coagulation (DIC)

7 y/o with h/o viral URI 1 week ago presents with epistaxis; PE: petechial hemorrhages of nasal mucosa and extremities; W/U: ↓ platelets, normal PT and PTT; bone marrow biopsy: ↑↑ megakaryocytes

Idiopathic thrombocytopenia purpura (ITP)

8 y/o with a h/o vomiting and diarrhea after eating a hamburger last week presents with fatigue, periorbital edema, and oliguria; PE: purpuric rash; CBC: ↓ platelets; PBS: burr cells, helmet cells; UA: RBC casts, proteinuria, hematuria

Hemolytic-uremic syndrome (HUS)

8 y/o with a h/o environmental allergies presents with a painful rash on the legs, abdominal discomfort, joint pain; UA: hematuria and RBC casts; Renal biopsy: glomerular mesangial IgA deposits

Henoch-Schönlein purpura

8 y/o male presents with a swollen painful knee; FH: maternal grandfather died from hemorrhage after a cholecystectomy; PE: cutaneous ecchymoses; W/U: gross blood in swollen knee joint, ↑ PTT, normal PT, platelet count, ↑ bleeding time

Hemophilia A

2 y/o male with a h/o recurrent epistaxis presents with the third episode of otitis media in 4 months; PE: eczematous dermatitis; W/U: thrombocytopenia, ↓ IgM, ↑ IgA

Wiskott-Aldrich syndrome

A newborn develops jaundice rapidly during the first day of life; PE: HSM; W/U: severe anemia, ⊕ indirect Coombs' test in both mother and newborn

Rh incompatibility

16 y/o female with a h/o menorrhagia presents with fatigue; PE: multiple cutaneous bruises; guaiac ⊕ stools; W/U: ↑ bleeding time, ↓ Factor VIII, normal platelet count, PT and PTT

von Willebrand's disease

RHEUMATOLOGY/MUSCULOSKELETAL

Spinal Disorders

Name the lower back condition associated with each of the following findings:

Saddle anesthesia with bowel/bladder dysfunction

Cauda equina syndrome

Positive "shopping-cart sign"

Spinal stenosis (patients more comfortable when leaning forward)

Increased pain at night that is unrelieved by positional changes or rest

Malignancy

Positive straight leg raise

Herniated disk → nerve root impingement

Increased pain with rest; pain improves with activity

Ankylosing spondylitis

Paraspinous muscle pain

Back strain (muscle) or sprain (ligamentous)

Pseudoclaudication, ↑ pain with walking

Spinal stenosis

Pain radiating from lower back down to the foot

Sciatica

Name four "red flags" of low back pain.

1. H/o malignancy
2. Constitutional symptoms (fever, weight loss)
3. Bladder/bowel dysfunction
4. Saddle anesthesia

What is the treatment for low back pain in the absence of "red flags"?

Conservative: NSAIDs/ acetaminophen, 1–3 days bed rest (85% resolve spontaneously)

What four chronic inflammatory conditions cause fusion of the sacroiliac joints?

The seronegative spondyloarthropathies: ankylosing spondylitis (AS), Reiter's syndrome, psoriatic arthritis, enteropathic arthritis

What haplotype is typically associated with the >90% of seronegative spondyloarthropathies?	HLA-B27

Joints

What is the definitive diagnostic procedure for acute monoarticular arthritis?	Arthrocentesis
Interpret each of the following arthrocentesis leukocyte counts (cells/mm^3):	
<200 WBCs	Normal joint fluid
<2000 WBCs	Noninflammatory (e.g., OA)
2000–50,000 WBCs	Mild-to-moderate inflammation (e.g., rheumatologic)
50,000–100,000 WBCs	Severe inflammation (e.g., septic arthritis or gout)
>100,000 WBCs	Septic joint (until proven otherwise)
What disease is characterized by monoarticular arthritis due to urate crystal deposits?	Gout
What are the two main etiologies of hyperuricemia?	1. Inadequate uric acid *excretion* (most of cases) 2. Uric acid *overproduction* (e.g., malignancy, hemolysis, LeschNyhan syndrome)
What is the most common presenting symptom?	Podogra (inflammation of first metatarsal-phalangeal [MTP] joint)
Why do tophi develop?	Chronic gout → deposits of urate crystals
Name the classic radiographic finding in advanced gout.	Classic "rat-bite" appearance to joint (punched-out erosion with overhanging cortical bone)
What does the joint fluid aspiration of gout reveal?	Needle-shaped, negatively-birefringent crystals under polarized light
What is the treatment for acute gout?	Colchicine and NSAIDs (e.g., indomethacin)

What is the maintenance therapy for gout?	**Overproducers** → allopurinol; **underexcreters** → probenecid/ sulfinpyrazone (**Note:** Continue colchicine because may precipitate acute attack)
What disease is characterized by calcium Pyrophosphate crystal deposition in joints?	Pseudogout
What does the joint fluid aspiration of pseudogout reveal?	Positively-birefringent crystals under polarized light
What chronic, systemic inflammatory arthritis is associated with HLA-DR4 serotype?	Rheumatoid arthritis (RA)

Name the seven diagnostic criteria for Rheumatoid authritis (RA)

1. Morning stiffness (>1 h)
2. Arthritis of three or more joints area (14 possible areas include R or L PIP, MCP, wrist, elbow, knee, ankle, and MTP joints)
3. Arthritis of one + hand joints (wrist, MCP, or PIP)
4. Symmetric arthritis
5. Rheumatoid nodules
6. ↑ serum RF—70% of cases
7. Radiographic changes: juxta-articular decalcification and late erosions

Note: 4 of 7 required to classify as RA

What is the term for the classic joint deformity associated with RA?	Boutonniere deformity

Name five extraarticular manifestations of RA.

1. Subcutaneous rheumatoid nodules
2. Asymptomatic pericardial effusions
3. Anemia of chronic disease
4. Nerve entrapment (e.g., carpal tunnel syndrome)
5. Pulmonary (effusions, interstitial fibrosis, nodule)

What is the treatment for RA?

Pain: First line = NSAIDs, then steroids; **disease-modifying**: first line = hydroxychloroquine, then MTX and biologic agents

Name two of the newer biologic agents used to treat RA.	Infliximab (anti-TNF-αAB) and Etanercept (anti-TNF receptor AB)
What syndrome is characterized by RA, splenomegaly, and leukopenia?	Felty's syndrome

Name the seronegative spondylarthropathy associated with the following statements:

Associated with sacroilitis	Ankylosing spondylarthritis
Precipitated by GI or GU infection	Reactive arthritis
Associated with nail pitting and DIP joint involvement	Psoriatic arthritis
Associated with inflammatory bowel disease	Enteropathic arthritis
What special type of reactive arthritis may be seen in HLA-B27 $\oplus$ males?	Reiter's syndrome
How does Reiter's syndrome typically present?	**"Can't SEE, can't PEE, can't CLIMB UP A TREE"** (conjunctivitis, urethritis, and arthritis)
Name two classic dermatologic findings of Reiter's syndrome.	Keratoderma blennorrhagicum and balanitis circinata
What is the treatment for Reiter's syndrome?	Erythromycin (for *Chlamydia*) and NSAIDs for arthritis; may benefit from prolonged tetracycline (3 months)

Osteoarthritis

Name the most common cause of arthritis.	Osteoarthritis (OA)
What noninflammatory arthritis is caused by wear and tear and is relieved by rest?	OA
Name three risk factors for OA.	Obesity, $\oplus$ FH, h/o joint trauma
Name three classic PE findings in OA.	Heberden's nodes (DIP), Bouchard nodes (PIP), and marked crepitus of affected joint
What is the classic radiographic appearance of OA?	Osteophytes and asymmetric joint space loss
What is the management of OA?	Isometric exercise to strengthen muscles at joint; NSAIDs (including cyclooxygenase [COX-2] inhibitors); joint replacement as last resort

Bones

Name the metabolic bone disease
associated with each of the following
statements:

Osteopenia with normal bone mineralization	Osteoporosis
Results from idiopathic hyperactivity of both osteoblasts and osteoclasts	Paget's bone disease (osteitis deformans)
$2°$ to vitamin D deficiency	Rickets (kids), osteomalacia (adults)
Vitamin C deficiency $\rightarrow \downarrow$ osteoid formation	Scurvy
Results from postmenopausal estrogen deficiency, physical inactivity, or calcium deficiency	Osteoporosis
Findings include Harrison groove, pigeon breast, craniotabes, and rachitic rosary	Rickets/osteomalacia
Findings include bleeding gums and "woody leg"	Scurvy
Findings include bone pain, deafness, and high-output cardiac failure	Paget's bone disease (osteitis deformans)
Dual energy x-ray absorptiometry (DEXA) scan shows significantly $\downarrow$ bone density	Osteoporosis
$\uparrow$ ALP; sclerotic lesions on XR	Paget's bone disease (osteitis deformans)
Death or decay of bone due to local ischemia in the absence of infection	Avascular necrosis (AVN)
Name five risk factors for osteoporosis.	Menopause, smoking, low body weight, long-term heparin or glucocorticoid use, alcoholism
What are the treatment options for senile (postmenopausal) osteoporosis?	Most important is prevention; treatment options: estrogen replacement (the only treatment shown to $\uparrow$ bone growth), Ca^{2+}, vitamin D, exercise); second line = bisphosphonates and calcitonin
What is the treatment for Paget's bone disease?	First line = bisphosphonates; second line = calcitonin

What bone disease is characterized by idiopathic replacement of bone with fibrous tissue?	Fibrous dysplasia
What syndrome is characterized by polyostotic fibrous dysplasia, precocious puberty, and café-au-lait spots?	McCune-Albright syndrome
What pediatric disease is characterized by the triad of skull lesions, DI, and exophthalmos?	Hand-Schüller-Christian disease
What is the most common primary malignant tumor of bone?	Osteosarcoma
Where does osteosarcoma typically occur?	Distal femur and proximal tibia
What is the classic radiographic appearance?	"Sunburst" sign (lytic lesion with spiculated periostitis) and Codman's triangle

Fractures and Dislocations

See Chapter 2: Surgery-Orthopedics

Muscle Diseases

Name the two major categories of muscle diseases.	1. **Neurogenic** (no pain, distal weakness, $\oplus$ fasciculations) 2. **Myopathic** (often painful, proximal weakness, no fasciculations)
Name the specific skeletal muscle disease associated with the following clinical and pathologic findings:	
Anti-ACh receptor ABs; associated with thymomas and autoimmune disorders	Myasthenia gravis
Most common and most lethal muscular dystrophy	Duchenne's muscular dystrophy
X-linked disease caused by a variety of mutations → ↓ functional dystrophin	Becker's muscular dystrophy
Paraneoplastic disorder commonly seen in patients with small cell carcinoma of the lung	Lambert-Eaton syndrome

Decreasing muscle strength with repetitive nerve stimulation	Myasthenia gravis
Muscular disorder associated with gonadal atrophy, baldness, cataracts, cardiomyopathy, and ↓ IgG	Myotonic dystrophy
Antibodies to presynaptic Ca^{2+} channels; ↑ muscle strength with repetitive nerve stimulation	Lambert-Eaton Syndrome
Progressive X-linked disease causing deficiency of dystrophin	Duchenne muscular dystrophy
Variable muscle weakness, most pronounced in occular and facial muscles initially	Myasthenia gravis
Painful, autoinflammatory disorder causing progressive, symmetric muscle weakness, dysphonia, and ↑ serum CPK	Polymyositis
Calf pseudohypertrophy and Gower sign	Duchenne muscular dystrophy
Gait instability (due to weakness of foot dorsiflexion) and involuntary muscle contraction on examination	Myotonic dystrophy

Name the muscle tumor associated with each of the following statements:

Most common tumor in females; estrogen sensitive → may grow during pregnancy and regress during menopause	Leiomyoma
Aggressive, malignant tumor of skeletal muscle; one of the small, round, blue cell tumors of childhood	Rhabdomyosarcoma

Rheumatology

Describe the effect(s) of SLE on each of the following organs:

Skin	Malar rash, discoid rash, photosensitivity
Joints	Arthritis and arthralgia
Central nervous system	Neuropsychiatric changes or seizures (2° to cerebral vasculitis)

Heart	Pericarditis, Libman-Sacks endocarditis (SLE→*LSE*)
Lungs	Pleuritis, pulmonary fibrosis
GI	Oral and nasopharyngeal ulcers
Kidneys	Wire-loop glomerular lesions and mesangial immune complex deposits → glomerulonephritis
Hematology	Hemolytic anemia, leukopenia, thrombocytopenia, Raynaud's phenomena
What pathologic finding is common to all tissues affected by SLE?	Acute necrotizing vasculitis of small arteries and arterioles caused by immune complex deposition
Libman-Sacks endocarditis causes sterile vegetations to form on both sides of which cardiac valve?	Mitral valve
Name five medications capable of inducing a lupus-like syndrome.	Hydralazine, INH, phenytoin, procainamide, penicillamine
Name the disease related to SLE that is characterized by immune complex deposition at the dermal-epidermal junction.	Discoid lupus erythematosus

Describe the disease associated with the following autoantibodies:

ANA (antinuclear antibodies)	SLE (sensitive but not specific for SLE)
Anti-ACh (acetylcholine)	Myasthenia gravis
Antibasement membrane	Goodpasture's disease
Anticentromere	**CREST** syndrome (**C**alcinosis, **R**aynaud's, **E**sophageal dysmotility, **S**clerodactyly, **T**elangiectasias)
Anti-dsDNA	SLE (highly specific for SLE)
Antiepithelial cell	Pemphigus vulgaris
Antigliadin	Celiac sprue
Antihistone	Drug-induced lupus erythematosus
Anti-IgG Fc	RA (RF factor)
Anti-Jo1	Myositis
Antimicrosomal	Hashimoto's thyroiditis
Antimitochondrial	Primary biliary cirrhosis

Anti-nRNP (nuclear ribonucleoprotein)	Mixed connective tissue disease
Antiplatelet	ITP
Anti-Scl-70 (DNA topoisomerase 1)	Diffuse scleroderma
Anti-Smith	SLE (highly specific for SLE)
Anti-SS-A (Ro) and anti-SS-B (La)	Sjögren syndrome
Antithyroglobulin	Hashimoto's thyroiditis
Anti-TSHr (TSH receptor)	Graves' disease
C-ANCA	Wegener's granulomatosis
Perinuclear pattern of antineutrophil cytoplasmic antibodies (P-ANCA)	Micropolyarteritis nodosa (PAN) and Churg-Strauss

Name the autoimmune disease of connective tissue associated with the following clinical and pathologic findings:

Keratoconjunctivitis sicca or xerophthalmia, xerostomia, and evidence of other connective tissue disease	Sjögren syndrome
Myositis and heliotrope rash	Dermatomyositis
Rapidly progressive diffuse fibrosis of skin and involved organs including the heart, GI tract, kidney, lung, muscle, and skin	Diffuse scleroderma
CREST syndrome	Localized scleroderma
Disease of connective tissue that lacks renal involvement	Mixed connective tissue disease

What is the most common cause of death due to scleroderma?	Renal crisis (occurs in 50% deaths from scleroderma; treat with ACE inhibitors)
Name the group of disorders characterized by extracellular deposition of protein in a β-pleated sheet conformation.	Amyloidosis (birefringence with Congo Red stain)

Name the effect of amyloidosis on each of the following organs:

Kidneys	Glomerular, peritubular, and vascular hyalinization

Liver	Hepatomegaly (amyloid deposition in space of Disse)
Heart	Restrictive cardiomyopathy
Tongue	Hypertrophy due to amyloid deposition

Make the Diagnosis

25 y/o male presents with morning stiffness, heel pain, and photophobia; PE: ↓ lumbar spine extension and lateral flexion, tenderness over lumbar spinous processes and iliac crests; W/U: HLA-B27 ⊕; XR: bamboo spine	Ankylosing spondylitis
50 y/o female presents with long-standing h/o morning stiffness and diffuse joint pain; PE: boutonierre and swan neck deformities of fingers, shoulder tenderness and ↓ range of motion (ROM), symmetric and bilateral knee swelling; W/U: RF ⊕	Rheumatoid arthritis (RA)
25 y/o male with a h/o urethritis 2 weeks ago presents with unilateral knee pain, stiffness, and eye pain; PE: conjunctivitis, edema and tenderness of left knee, mucoid urethral discharge; W/U: urethral swab is ⊕ for *Chlamydia*	Reiter's syndrome
45 y/o female presents with dry eyes and dry mouth, PE: parotid gland enlargement; W/U: ⊕ ANA, RF, SS-A/Ro titers	Sjögren syndrome
70 y/o female presents with pain in hands that is worse after activity; PE: Heberden's nodes and Bouchard's nodes, bony enlargement at DIP joints, right knee effusion; W/U: RF and ESR are WNL; XR: joint space narrowing, osteophytes	Osteoarthritis (OA)
72 y/o female presents with a 6-week. h/o morning stiffness in neck and shoulders; PE: low-grade fever, tenderness to palpation plus ↓ ROM in neck, shoulder, and hip joints; W/U: ↑ ESR, CRP, RF negative	Polymyalgia rheumatica

50 y/o male presents with acute onset of sharp pain in the left great toe; PE: severe tenderness, swelling, and warmth of the left MTP joint; Synovial fluid analysis shows negatively-birefringent crystals	Gout
25 y/o Black female with a 1 week h/o pain in several joints presents with swelling, redness, and pain in her right knee; PE: pustular lesions on palms, right knee shows erythema, tenderness, and ↓ ROM; W/U: Gram negative diplococci in synovial fluid	Gonococcal arthritis
28 y/o female presents with difficulty keeping her eyelids open and holding her head up during the day; PE: weakness of facial muscles, deltoids; ⊕ anti-ACh titer; CXR: anterior mediastinal mass	Myasthenia gravis (associated with thymoma)
25 y/o female with h/o Raynaud's phenomenon presents with arthralgias and myositis; WU: esophageal hypomotility and ↑ anti-nRNP titers	Mixed connective tissue disease
20 y/o Black female presents with fatigue, arthralgias, Raynaud's phenomenon, and pleuritic chest pain; PE: butterfly malar facial rash; W/U: ↓ platelets, proteinuria, and ⊕ ANA, anti-dsDNA, and anti-Smith ABs	SLE
20 y/o with a h/o developmental delay presents with facial weakness; PE: cataracts, marked weakness in muscles of hand, neck, and distal leg, with sustained muscle contraction; Genetic testing: CTG repeat expansion within DMPK gene	Myotonic dystrophy

DERMATOLOGY

Basic Vocabulary

Give the dermatologic term for
each of the following descriptions:

Flat, nonpalpable lesion <1 cm in diameter; different colors that surround skin	Macule

A macule >1 cm in diameter	Patch
Palpable, elevated skin lesion <1 cm in diameter	Papule
A papule >1 cm in diameter	Plaque
Minute, pinpoint, nonblanching hemorrhagic spots in the skin	Petechiae
Similar to petechiae, but larger	Purpura
Fluid-containing blister <0.5 cm in diameter	Vesicle
Fluid-containing blister >0.5 cm in diameter	Bulla
Blister containing pus	Pustule
Solid, round lesion; diameter = thickness	Nodule
Leathery induration of skin caused by scratching	Lichenification
Thickening of the stratum corneum	Hyperkeratosis

Infections

For each of the following descriptions, name the lesion and the treatment of choice:

Inflammation of pilosebaceous unit by *Propionibacterium,* causing comedones and pustules; ↑ during puberty and adolescence	Acne vulgaris **Tx** = Topical antibiotics, Retin-A, benzoyl peroxide, isotretinoin if scarring
Honey-colored, crusty vesicles commonly occurring around the mouth and nose in children; caused by *Staphylococcus aureus* or *Streptococcus pyogenes*	Impetigo **Tx** = Wash with warm cloth; keflex or oxacillin for 7–10 days
Subcutaneous, soft-tissue infection with classic signs of inflammation; caused by *Staphylococcus aureus* or *Streptococcus pyogenes*	Cellulitis **Tx** = Keflex or dicloxacillin for 7–10 days
Erythematous rash along major skin folds; more common in diabetics; caused by *Corynebacterium*	**Erythr**asma **Tx** = **Erythr**omycin

Umbilicated, pearly, dome-shaped papules typically occurring in the genitals; viral etiology	Molluscum contagiosum **Tx** = Cryotherapy or trichloroacetic acid (many resolve spontaneously without treatment)
Tender red nodules on the anterior tibial area bilaterally $2°$ to panniculitis; due to infections, drugs, or inflammatory bowel disease	Erythema nodosum **Tx** = NSAIDs; treat underlying cause
"Sunburn with goosebumps" appearance, Pastia line, strawberry tongue; caused by *S. pyogenes*	Scarlet fever **Tx** = Penicillin
Small pink papules in groups of 10–20 on the trunk; found in 30% of patients with *Salmonella typhi*	Rose spots **Tx** = Cholecystectomy for chronic carrier state
Suppurative inflammation of the nail fold surrounding the nail plate; may be due to staphylococci and streptococci infection	Paronychia **Tx** = Warm compress; Keflex if severe
Infection along a fascial plane causing severe pain and inflammation; caused by *S. pyogenes* or *C. perfringens*	Necrotizing fasciitis **Tx** = Extensive surgical debridement plus clindamycin and penicillin
Obstructed apocrine sweat glands that become infected	Hidradenitis suppurativa **Tx** = Surgical debridement and antibiotics
Recurrent, vesicular eruption that occur in groups and are painful; commonly found at oral-labial or genital locations; diagnose with Tzanck smear	Herpes simplex **Tx** = Oral acyclovir (IV if immunocompromised)
Benign papilloma of viral etiology, most commonly on dorsum of hand; characteristic koilocytes	Verruca vulgaris (common wart) **Tx** = Cryotherapy or salicylic acid
Contagious, pruritic, "dewdrop" vesicles that occur in kids and can be reactivated into a painful, dermatomal distribution in adults	Varicella (chickenpox and shingles) **Tx** = Acyclovir for shingles; self-limited in healthy kids; varicella vaccine available for immunocompromised
Pruritic papules in pubic area, buttocks, and axilla caused by lice	Crabs (Pediculosis pubis) **Tx** = Permethrin 5% shampoo

Contagious, erythematous, pruritic papules, and burrows in intertriginous areas caused by mites	Scabies (Sarcoptes scabiei) Tx = Permethrin 5% cream for patient and close contacts; wash bedding with hot water
Ring-shaped, pruritic, erythematous plaque with elevated borders; caused by fungus	Tinea (corporis if on body; capitis if on head) Tx = Topical antifungal; oral for tinea capitis or resistant lesions
Erythematous scaling patches with satellite pustules, found in intertriginous areas of adults and diaper areas in infants	*Candida* Tx = Reduce moisture; topical nystatin
Sharply demarcated, *hypopigmented* macules with characteristic "spaghetti and meatball" appearance on KOH prep	Tinea versicolor Tx = Selenium sulfide shampoo or topical antifungal

Pigmentary Lesions

Name the dermatologic disease or finding associated with each of the following descriptions:

AR defect in melanin synthesis (though melanocytes are present); predisposition to multiple skin disorders	Albinism (oculocutaneous)
Acquired loss of melanocytes → depigmented white patches	Vitiligo
Mask-like facial hyperpigmentation associated with pregnancy	Melasma (chloasma)
Pigmented macules caused by melanocyte hyperplasia; do not darken with sunlight (unlike freckles)	Lentigo
Benign, localized overgrowth of melanin-forming cells of the skin present at birth	Nevocellular nevus
Atypical, irregularly pigmented lesion may evolve into malignant melanoma	Dysplastic nevus
Common benign neoplasm of older adults; sharply demarcated plaques with a pasted on appearance	Seborrheic keratosis (senile keratosis)

Yellowish papules or nodules that tend to occur on the eyelids; associated with hypercholesterolemia	Xanthoma (on the eyelids = xanthelasma)
Hyperpigmentation in the flexural areas that may suggest visceral malignancy	Acanthosis nigricans
Abnormal proliferation of connective tissue that may follow skin trauma; results in large, raised tumor-like scar	Keloid
Capillary hemangioma appearing as a purple-red area on the face or neck	Port-wine stain
Autoimmune disorder presenting with heliotropic patches on eyelids	Dermatomyositis
Erythematous rash that can appear in Christmas tree distribution and is preceded by a herald patch	Pityriasis rosea
Hyperpigmentation, cirrhosis, diabetes mellitus, OA of MCP joints	Hemochromatosis

Name the neurocutaneous syndrome characterized by each of the following features:

Port-wine stains of the face, ipsilateral glaucoma, retinal lesions, and hemangiomas of the meninges	Sturge-Weber syndrome
Hypopigmented macules (ash-leaf spots), adenoma sebaceum, seizures, and mental retardation	Tuberous sclerosis
Multiple organ hemangioblastomas, cysts, and paragangliomas	von Hippel-Lindau disease
Café-au-lait spots, acoustic neuromas, and meningiomas	Neurofibromatosis

Miscellaneous Dermatologic Diseases

Name the blistering dermal disease associated with each of the following descriptions:

Tense, hard subepidermal bullae that tend to occur in the elderly; antiepidermal BM Abs	Bullous pemphigoid

Pruritic subepidermal blisters occurring in groups; eosinophils and IgA deposits at tips of dermal papillae; seen in celiac disease	Dermatitis herpetiformis
Large intraepidermal blisters that often rupture and slough off (Nikolsky's sign); can be fatal; antibodies to desmoglein	Pemphigus vulgaris
Hypersensitivity reaction causing characteristic diffuse, multishaped "target" lesions	Erythema multiforme
Severe-febrile form of erythema multiforme characterized by systemic toxicity, hemorrhagic crusting, and oral mucosal involvement	Stevens-Johnson syndrome
AD defect in heme synthesis; blisters on sun-exposed areas of skin; urine fluoresces orange-pink color with Wood's lamp examination	Porphyria cutanea tarda
What inflammatory disorder is characterized by silvery scaling plaques over the knees, elbows, and scalp?	Psoriasis
Name three classic clinical findings in psoriasis.	1. Fingernail pitting 2. Auspitz sign (removal of scale causes pinpoint bleeding) 3. Koebner phenomenon (lesions appear at sites of cutaneous trauma)
What is the treatment of choice for psoriasis?	First line = topical steroids; second line = PUVA (Psoralens plus UVA light rays)

For each of the following descriptions, name the lesion and the treatment of choice:

Pruritic, inflammatory disorders due to an inherited state of hyper-sensitivity to environmental allergens	Atopic dermatitis Tx = Steroids/antihistamines for symptomatic relief
Linear, pruritic rash caused by type IV hypersensitivity reaction to previously sensitized substance	Contact dermatitis Tx = Topical steroids; antihistamines and systemic steroids for severe cases

Greasy, erythematous scaling patches of the scalp, face, and ears; "cradle cap" in infants	Seborrheic dermatitis Tx = Selenium sulfide or zinc pyrithione shampoo for scalp, face, and trunk; steroids if severe
Intensely pruritic, transient, erythematous, papular wheals caused by mast cell degranulation and histamine release	Urticaria (hives) Tx = Steroids/antihistamines for symptomatic relief

Skin Cancer

Name the skin malignancy associated with each of the following statements:

Most common skin malignancy	Basal cell carcinoma
Associated with excessive sunlight exposure; arises from dysplastic nevus cells	Malignant melanoma
Associated with arsenic and radiation exposure	Squamous cell carcinoma
Actinic keratosis is a precursor	Squamous cell carcinoma
Pearly papule with translucent border and fine telangiectasias	Basal cell carcinoma
Small, exophytic nodule with crusting or scaling	Squamous cell carcinoma
S-100 used as a tumor marker	Malignant melanoma
Histopathology characterized by "keratin pearls"	Squamous cell carcinoma
Characterized by radial and vertical growth phases	Malignant melanoma
Characterized by locally aggressive, ulcerating, and hemorrhagic lesions; almost never metastatic	Basal cell carcinoma
Occurs in sun-exposed areas and tends to involve the **lower** part of the face	Squamous cell carcinoma
Occurs in sun-exposed areas and tends to involve the **upper** part of the face	Basal cell carcinoma
What is management for actinic keratosis?	Biopsy; treatment with topical 5-fluorouracil (5-FU) or cryotherapy; prevention with sunscreens

Name the ABCDE characteristics of melanomas.	Asymmetry (benign is symmetric)
	Border (benign is smooth)
	Color (benign is single color)
	Diameter (benign is <6 mm)
	Elevation (benign is flat) and
	Enlargement (benign is not growing)
What is the most important prognostic factor in malignant melanoma?	Depth of invasion
What clinical variant of malignant melanoma has the poorest prognosis?	Nodular melanoma
What clinical variant of malignant melanoma often appears on the hands and feet of dark-skinned people?	Acral-lentiginous melanoma
What chronic progressive lymphoma arises in the skin and initially simulates eczema?	Mycosis fungoides
What syndrome is characterized by mycosis fungoides, erythroderma, and scaling?	Sézary syndrome
What connective tissue cancer presents with reddish-purple macules, plaques, or nodules on the skin and mucosa and is caused by HHV-8?	Kaposi's sarcoma

Name the classic dermatologic finding(s) associated with each of the following diseases:

Gastric adenocarcinoma	Acanthosis nigricans
Addison's disease	Hyperpigmentation and striae
Rheumatic fever	Erythema marginatum
Kawasaki syndrome	Erythematous palms and soles; dry, red lips; desquamation of fingertips
Severe chronic renal failure	Uremic frost
Bacterial endocarditis	Osler's nodes (tender, raised lesions on pads of fingers or toes) and Janeway lesions (small, erythematous lesions on palms or soles)
Xeroderma pigmentosum	Dry skin and melanoma
Hypothyroidism	Cool, dry skin with coarse brittle hair
Graves' disease	Warm, moist skin with fine hair; pretibial myxedema

von Recklinghausen's disease (NFT1)	Multiple
Familial hypercholesterolemia	Xanthom
SLE	Malar ra:
Pellagra	Dermatit

Name the classic dermatologic finding(s) associated with each of the following infectious diseases:

Anthrax	Vesicular papules covered by black eschar
Parvovirus B$_{19}$	Erythema infectiosum (*slapped-cheek* appearance)
Lyme disease	Erythema chronicum migrans
Primary syphilis	Painless chancre
Secondary syphilis	Rash over palms and soles, condyloma latum
Rocky mountain spotted fever (RMSF)	Rash over palms and soles (migrates centrally)
Congenital CMV	Pinpoint petechial "blueberry muffin" rash
HPV (in genital region)	Condylomata acuminata
Leprosy	Hypopigmented, anesthetic skin patches

Make the Diagnosis

30 y/o male with h/o recurrent sinusitis presents for sterility evaluation; PE: heart sounds are best heard over right side of chest	Kartagener syndrome
9 y/o with h/o easy bruising and hyperextensible joints presents to the ER after dislocating his shoulder for the fifth time this year	Ehlers-Danlos syndrome
5 y/o presents to the ER with his sixth bone fracture in the past 2 years; PE: bluish sclera and mild kyphosis; XR: fractures with evidence of osteopenia	Osteogenesis imperfecta (OI)
8 y/o with h/o severe sunburns and photophobia presents to the dermatologist for evaluation of several lesions on the face that have recently changed color and size	Xeroderma pigmentosum

resents to the ophthalmology th sudden ↓ visual acuity; PE: al body habitus, long and slender ers, pectus excavatum, and superiorly slocated lens	Marfan syndrome
36 y/o with h/o celiac disease presents with clusters of erythematous vesicular lesions over the extensor surfaces of the extremities	Dermatitis herpetiformis
5 y/o patient presents with honey-colored crusted lesions at the angle of his mouth; Gram stain of pus: gram-positive cocci in chains	Impetigo
29 y/o HIV ⊕ patient presents with multiple painless pearly-white umbilicated nodules on the trunk and anogenital area	Molluscum contagiosum
68 y/o fair-skinned farmer presents with large, telangiectatic, and ulcerated nodule on the bridge of the nose	Basal cell carcinoma
11 y/o presents with bilateral wrist pain and a rash; PE: erythematous, reticular skin rash of the face and trunk with a "slapped-cheek appearance"	Erythema infectiosum
43 y/o female presents with difficulty swallowing; PE: bluish discoloration of the hands and shiny, tight skin over her face and fingers	Progressive systemic sclerosis (scleroderma)
5 y/o Asian boy presents with fever and diffuse rash including the palms and soles; PE: cervical lymphadenopathy, conjunctival injection, and desquamation of his fingertips; Echocardiogram reveals dilation of coronary arteries	Kawasaki syndrome (mucocutaneous lymph node syndrome)
33 y/o patient presents with itchy, purple plaques over her wrists, forearms, and inner thigh; PE: Wickham striae	Lichen planus
10 y/o presents with fevers and pruritic rash spreading from the trunk to the arms; PE: "teardrop"-shaped vesicles of varying stages	Varicella
29 y/o athlete presents with a red, pruritic skin eruption with an advancing peripheral, creeping border on the forearm; W/U: septate hyphae on KOH scraping	Tinea corporis (ringworm)

73 y/o presents with a painful, unilateral, vesicular rash in the distribution of the CN V$_1$; PE: diminished corneal sensation	Herpes zoster ophthalmicus
31 y/o obese female presents with pruritis in her skin folds; PE: white curd-like concretions beneath the abdominal panniculus; W/U shows budding yeast on 10% KOH prep	Cutaneous candidiasis

PREVENTATIVE MEDICINE, ETHICS, AND BIOSTATISTICS

Preventative Medicine

Describe the appropriate screening intervention for each of the following cancers:

Breast cancer	Self breast examination every month, >20 y/o
	Clinician breast examination every 3 years from 20 to 40 and every year >40 y/o
	Mammography every year from 50 to 69 y/o
Colon cancer	Hemoccult every year >50 y/o
	Flexible sigmoidoscopy every 3–5 years >50 y/o, *or* colonoscopy every 10 years
	Note: If ⊕ FH, start screening 10 years before age of family member with CA at diagnosis
Prostate cancer	DRE and PSA every year >50 y/o
Endometrial cancer	High-risk patients should be offered biopsy starting at 35 y/o
Cervical cancer	First pap smear by 3 years after sexual activity or 21 y/o; then every year thereafter
	At 30 y/o, after 3 consecutive normal paps → every 2–3 years
	Pelvic examination every 1–3 years from 20 to 40 and every year >40 y/o

**Name the adult immunization recommen-
dations for each of the following diseases:**

Varicella	Adults without h/o chickenpox or high-risk patients (e.g., immunocompromised)
Hepatitis B	All young adults and high-risk patients (including health care workers)
Pneumococcal	Administer once to patients >65 y/o or those at high risk
Influenza	Annually for patients >50 y/o or those at high risk
Meningococcal	High-risk patients (e.g., college students, military personnel)
Measles, mumps, rubella (MMR)	Everyone born after 1956 who has not yet received vaccination
Tetanus	Primary vaccination necessary for everyone; booster indicated every 10 years
Hepatitis A	Travelers, homosexual males, h/o chronic liver disease or clotting disorder (**Note:** Vaccination takes 3–4 weeks; give IVIG for short-term prophylaxis or h/o exposure)

What vaccines should be avoided in HIV⊕ and pregnant patients?

Live vaccinations (MMR, oral polio vaccine [OPV], VZV); **Note:** MMR should be given if CD4 >500

What is the regimen of choice for smoking cessation?

Bupropion plus nicotine replacement (12 months abstinence rate >30%; 2× >than nicotine alone)

Aging, Death, and Dying

Name the changes found in the elderly in each of the following categories:

Psychiatric	Depression and anxiety more common; suicide rate increases
Sexual	Men: Slower erection/ejaculation, ↑ refractory period Women: Vaginal shortening, thinning, and dryness

	Note: Sexual interest does NOT decrease
Sleep patterns	↓ REM, slow-wave sleep; ↑ sleep latency, awakenings
Cognitive	↓ learning speed; intelligence stays the same
Name three conditions that would qualify normal bereavement as pathologic grief.	1. Prolonged grief (>1 year) 2. Excessively intense grief (sleep disturbances, significant weight loss, suicidal ideations) 3. Grief that is delayed, inhibited, or denied
Name the Kübler-Ross stages of dying.	Denial, Anger, Bargaining, Depression, Acceptance (**Note:** One or more stages can occur at once and not necessarily in this order)
What term describes a centralized program of palliative and supportive services to dying persons and their families, in the form of physical, psychologic, social, and spiritual care?	Hospice
What are the criteria to qualify for this type of care?	Medically anticipated death within 6 months

Medical Ethics

Name the term used to describe each of the following ethical responsibilities:	
Requires physicians to "do no harm"	Nonmaleficence
Requires physicians to act in the best interests of the patient	Beneficence (may conflict with patient autonomy)
Demands respect for patient privacy and autonomy	Confidentiality
Name two situations in which a physician must compromise patient confidentiality.	1. Potential harm to self (suicide) or to a third party (Tarasoff decision) 2. Legally defined situations (e.g., reportable diseases, gunshot wounds, impaired drivers)
What elements are required in order to prove a malpractice claim?	The "**4 Ds**": Must prove that the physician showed **d**eriliction (deviation from standard of care) of a **d**uty that caused **d**amages **d**irectly to the patient

What are the four key components to informed consent?

The patient must:
1. Understand the health implications of their diagnosis
2. Be informed of risks, benefits, and alternatives to treatment
3. Be aware of outcome if they do not consent
4. Have the right to withdraw consent at any time

Name four exceptions to informed consent.

1. Patient not legally competent to make decisions
2. In an emergency (implied consent)
3. Patient waives the right to informed consent
4. Therapeutic privilege—withholding information that would severely harm the patient or undermine decision-making capacity if revealed

What are five situations in which parent/legal guardian consent is not required to treat a minor?

1. Emergencies
2. STDs
3. Prescription of contraceptives
4. Treatment of ETOH/drug treatment
5. Care during pregnancy

What four criteria qualify a minor as emancipated?

If minor is self-supporting, in the military, married, or a parent supporting children

What type of directive is based on the incapacitated patient's prior statements and decisions?

Oral advance directive (substituted judgment standard)

What written advance directive gives instructions for the patient's future health care should he/she become incompetent to make decisions?

Living will; specific examples include DNR (do not resuscitate) or DNI (do not intubate)

What document allows the patient to designate a surrogate to make medical decisions in case the patient loses decision-making capacity?

Durable power of attorney (more flexible than a living will)

When are physicians permitted to refuse a family's request for further intervention on behalf of an ill patient?

On grounds of futility (e.g., maximal intervention is failing, no rationale for treatment, and treatment will not achieve the goals of care)

Biostatistics and Clinical Trials

For each description, name the proper term and the equation used to calculate the value:

Probability that a person without the disease will be correctly identified	Specificity = TN/(TN + FP)
Probability that a person who tests positive actually has the disease	Positive predictive value = TP/(TP + FP)
Probability that a person who has a disease will be correctly identified	Sensitivity = TP/(TP + FN)
Total number of cases in a population at any given time	Prevalence = TP + FN/(entire population)
Number of new cases that arise in a population over a given time interval	Incidence= Prevalence × duration of disease (approximately)
Used in case-control studies to approximate the relative risk if the disease prevalence is too high	Odds ratio = TP x TN/FP x FN
Used in cohort studies to compare incidence rate in exposed group to that in unexposed group	Relative risk = [TP/(TP + FP)]/[FN/(FN + TN)]
Probability that patient with a negative test actually has no disease	Negative predictive value = TN/(FN + TN)
How are incidence and prevalence related?	Incidence × disease duration → prevalence
	Prevalence >incidence for chronic diseases; prevalence = incidence for acute diseases
What quality is desirable for a screening tool?	High sensitivity (**SNOUT** - **SeN**sitivity rules **OUT**)
What quality is desirable for a confirmatory test?	High specificity (**SPIN** - **SP**ecificity rules **IN**)
What is the term for a situation where one outcome is more likely to occur than another?	Bias
Name four ways to reduce bias.	1. Placebo 2. Blinded studies (single, double) 3. Crossover studies (each subject is own control) 4. Randomization

Name the type of study:

Observational study where the sample is chosen based on presence/absence of risk factors	Cohort study (e.g., prospective → provides relative risk)
Survey of a population at a single point in time; allows for estimate of disease prevalence	Cross-sectional survey
Experimental study comparing benefits of two or more alternative treatments	Clinical trial
Observational study where the sample is chosen based on disease presence/absence	Case-control study (usually retrospective) → provides odds ratio
Assembling data from multiple studies to achieve great statistical power	Metaanalysis

Name the term for each of the following descriptions:

Refers to the reproducibility of a test	Reliability
Refers to the appropriateness of a test (whether the test measures what it is supposed to)	Validity
Absence of random variation in a test; consistency and reproducibility of a test	Precision
Closeness of a measurement to the truth	Accuracy
Hypothesis postulating that there is no difference between groups	Null hypothesis (H_0)
Error of mistakenly rejecting H_0 (stating that there is a difference when there really is not)	Type I error (α)
Error of failing to reject H_0 (stating there is no difference when there really is)	Type II error (β)
Probability of rejecting H_0 when it is in fact false	Power ($1 - \beta$)
Probability of making an α error	P value
Test that compares the difference between two means	t test

Test that analyzes the variance of three or more variables	Analysis of variance (ANOVA)
Test that compares percentages or proportions	χ^2
Absolute value that indicates the strength of a relationship	r (always between -1 and 1)

Name the type of bias described in each of the following examples:

Responses to subjective questions are influenced by knowing what leg of the study a patient is enrolled	Observational bias
Confounding variables introduced by errors of memory made by participants asked to remember past events	Recall bias
Occurs when subjects are assigned to a study group in a nonrandom fashion	Enrollment bias
Bias that is dependent on the rate of disease progression; may lead to overestimation of screening effectiveness is disease	Length bias
Occurs when a patient chooses to enroll in a particular study	Self-selection bias
Occurs when screening tends to prolong the time between diagnosis and death without actually affecting true survival	Lead-time bias

Epidemiology

What is the leading cause of mortality in each of the following age groups:

<1 y/o	Congenital anomalies
1–14 years old	Unintentional injuries
15–24 years old	Unintentional injuries (mostly car accidents)
25–64 years old	Cancer (#1 lung, #2 breast/prostate, #3 colon)
65 years and older	In the appendix

CHAPTER 2

Surgery

TRAUMA

Shock

Define shock.	Inadequate tissue perfusion
What are the four main types of shock?	1. Cardiogenic 2. Septic 3. Hypovolemic 4. Neurogenic

Name the type of shock described below and give the appropriate management:

Hypotension, ↑ pulmonary capillary wedge pressure (PCWP), ↓ cardiac output (CO)	Cardiogenic (usually left ventricular failure) **Treatment/therapy (Tx):** Inotropic agents, afterload reduction
Tachycardia, ↓ systolic BP, and ↓ pulse pressure	Hypovolemic (usually hemorrhage or burns) **Tx:** IV fluid replacement with isotonic lactated Ringer's (LR) or normal saline (NS); controlling hemorrhage if applicable
Tachycardia, hypotension, ↑ CO, warm skin with full pulses, fever	Septic (usually secondary [2°] to gram-negative organisms) **Tx:** Aggressive IV fluids, antibiotics, vasopressors as needed
Hypotension and bradycardia	Neurogenic (loss of sympathetic tone) **Tx:** IV fluids and identification of neurologic deficits

What are the first five steps in the assessment of a trauma patient?	**A**irway: Secure airway while maintaining C-spine stability
	Breathing: Inspect for air movement, assess oxygenation, and ventilation
	Circulation: Assess pulses, heart rate, BP; secure IV access
	Disability: Diagnose neurologic deficits and estimate Glasgow Coma Scale (GCS)
	Exposure/environment: Complete visual inspection and palpation of patient while maintaining normal body temperature

Name the diagnosis associated with each of the following findings:

Hemotympanum, clear otorrhea/rhinorrhea, raccoon eyes, and Battle sign	Basilar skull fracture (Fx)
Ecchymosis of lower abdomen from seatbelt (seatbelt sign)	Small bowel perforation (in 20% of cases)
Hypotension, jugular venous distension (JVD), decreased heart sounds	Beck's triad (seen in cardiac tamponade, tension pneumothorax)
Beck triad and pulsus paradoxus	Cardiac tamponade
Unilateral absence of breath sounds, JVD, mediastinal shift	Tension pneumothorax
Paradoxical chest wall movement	Flail chest (multiple rib Fxs with pulmonary injury)

GENERAL SURGERY

Esophagus

What is the common presentation of *oropharyngeal* dysphagia?	Difficulty swallowing liquids > solids
What is the common presentation of *esophageal* dysphagia?	Difficulty swallowing *both* liquids and solids
What is the common presentation of dysphagia secondary to mechanical obstruction?	Difficulty swallowing solids > liquids

What is the differential diagnosis of oropharyngeal dysphagia? — Zenker's diverticulum, neurologic disorders (cranial nerves, muscles), sphincter dysfunction, and neoplasm

What term is used to describe a false diverticulum above the cricopharyngeus muscle? — Zenker's diverticulum

What two tests are essential in the evaluation of oropharyngeal dysphagia? — Barium swallow followed by endoscopy if no diverticulum is seen

What is the risk of endoscopy with oropharyngeal dysphagia? — Risk of esophageal perforation is high with Zenker's diverticulum. (Zenker's diverticulum must be ruled out with a barium swallow)

What is the treatment of a Zenker's diverticulum? — Myotomy ± excision of diverticulum

What is the differential diagnosis for esophageal dysphagia? —
1. Achalasia
2. Esophageal stricture
3. Lower esophageal web
4. Scleroderma
5. Esophageal cancer

Name the esophageal disease associated with the following characteristics:

Inability of the lower esophageal sphincter (LES) to relax with loss of esophageal persitalsis; "bird beak" appearance on barium swallow and $\uparrow$ resting pressure of LES on manometry — Achalasia (ganglionic loss of Auerbach's plexus)

May result from ingestion of caustic agents (e.g., lye, oven cleaners, batteries, or drain cleaners) — Esophageal stricture

Syndrome characterized by iron-deficiency anemia, dysphagia, esophageal web, and atrophic glossitis — Plummer-Vinson syndrome

Columnar metaplasia of squamous epithelium in distal esophagus in response to prolonged injury (often due to long-standing gastroesophageal reflux disease [GERD]) — Barrett's esophagus

What type of malignancy occurs in patients with long-standing Barrett's? — Esophageal cancer ($10\times \uparrow$ risk $\rightarrow$ rule out with endoscopy)

Name six important risk factors for esophageal carcinoma.

ABCDEF

Achalasia

Barrett's esophagus

Corrosive esophagitis

Diverticuli

Esophageal webs, ethanol (ETOH)

Familial

What are the two main histologic types of esophageal cancer?

Squamous cell carcinoma and adenocarcinoma near the gastroesophageal (GE) junction

What type of esophageal cancer is associated with alcohol and tobacco use?

Squamous cell carcinoma

Barrett's esophagus is a risk factor for what type of esophageal cancer?

Adenocarcinoma

What diagnostic test is necessary in the workup (W/U) for all patients with suspected esophageal cancer?

Esophagogastroduodenoscopy (EGD) with tissue biopsy

What diagnosis must be ruled out in a patient with the sudden onset of severe retrosternal chest pain worse with swallowing and deep inhalation following EGD?

Esophageal perforation

What syndrome is characterized by esophageal perforation following severe vomiting?

Boerhaave's syndrome

What term is used to describe the crunching sound heard with each heartbeat in a patient with mediastinal emphysema?

Hamman's sign

What tests are used to make a definitive diagnosis of esophageal perforation?

Chest x-ray (CXR) (showing mediastinal/subcutaneous air, pneumothorax, left pleural effusion) and esophagogram

What is the treatment of esophageal perforation?

Thoracotomy, primary repair, and drainage within 24 h (>50% mortality if treatment delayed)

What disease is characterized by substernal chest pain, heartburn, and regurgitation, commonly worse after meals and in the supine position?

GERD

Symptoms of what pulmonary condition may be seen in patients with GERD?

Asthma (wheezing/cough/dyspnea)

Name the six major risk factors for GERD.	1. Obesity 2. Pregnancy 3. Alcohol 4. Caffeine 5. Smoking 6. Fatty food diet
Name three diseases closely associated with GERD.	Sliding hiatal hernia, scleroderma, and achalasia
Name three diagnostic studies that can be used to make a diagnosis of GERD.	1. EGD 2. pH probe 3. Barium swallow
What condition is a major concern in patients with long-standing GERD?	Barrett's esophagus (metaplasia of distal esophagus)
What is the medical treatment for Barrett's esophagus?	Antacids, H_2 blockers, or proton pump inhibitors (PPi) with surveillance EGD and biopsies
Name five possible complications of GERD.	1. Ulceration 2. Stricture formation 3. Barrett's esophagus 4. Bleeding 5. Aspiration of gastric contents
What are the indications for surgery in a patient with GERD?	Failure of medical treatment, stricture formation, severe dyphasia, Barrett's esophagus

Stomach

What disease is characterized by erosion of the gastric or duodenal mucosa?	Peptic ulcer disease (PUD)
What are the classic symptoms associated with PUD?	Epigastric pain relieved with antacids, nausea, "coffee-ground" emesis, melena, or hematochezia
What is the differential diagnosis of epigastric pain?	1. PUD 2. Gastritis 3. Pancreatitis 4. Cholecystitis 5. Coronary artery disease (CAD) 6. GERD
What pathogen is found in >90% of patients with duodenal ulcers and 70% of patients with gastric ulcer disease?	*Helicobacter pylori*
Aside from *H. pylori* infection, name three other common risk factors for PUD.	NSAIDs, ETOH, and smoking

What study is used to definitively diagnose PUD?	EGD with biopsies (for *H. pylori* and to rule out gastric cancer)
What is the most common location of a *gastric* ulcer?	Body of the stomach
What is the most common location of a *duodenal* ulcer?	First part of the duodenum

Name the type of peptic ulcer (gastric or duodenal) associated with each of the following findings:

Pain is worse during meals	Gastric ulcer (pain is **G**reater with meals) → weight loss
Pain improves after meals	Duodenal ulcer (pain **D**ecreases with meals) → weight gain
Almost 100% associated with *H. pylori* infection	Duodenal ulcer
NSAIDs, alcohol use, and smoking are implicated in pathogenesis	Gastric ulcer
Gastric acid production may be reduced	Gastric ulcer
Associated with Zollinger-Ellison syndrome; ↑ serum gastrin levels	Duodenal ulcer
Most common type of PUD	Duodenal ulcer (twice as common as gastric ulcers)
Occur in the setting of ↓ mucosal protection against gastric acid	Both
What are the four treatment goals for PUD?	1. Decrease acid production 2. Mucosal protection 3. Eradication of *H. pylori* 4. Cancer surveillance (gastric)
What medications are used for acid suppression?	H_2 blockers and PPi
What medications are used for mucosal protection?	Sucralfate, bismuth, and misoprostol
What is the treatment for *H. pylori*?	"Triple therapy" (PPi, bismuth salicylate, and two of the following antibiotics: metronidazole, amoxicillin, clarithromycin, or tetracycline); requires 6–8 weeks to heal

What diagnostic study must be performed in patients with nonhealing gastric ulcers?

EGD with biopsy

Name three common complications of PUD requiring intervention.

1. Hemorrhage from erosion of an ulcer into a blood vessel
2. Perforation
3. Obstruction

What are the classic symptoms of gastric outlet obstruction?

Nausea/vomiting (N/V), crampy abdominal pain, weight loss, and distented/dilated stomach

What is the typical presentation of a perforated ulcer?

Sudden, severe onset abdominal pain radiating to back and shoulders, N/V, and peritoneal signs (rebound tenderness, guarding, and motion pain on examination)

What finding on x-ray is an absolute indication for surgery?

Free air under the diaphragm

What is the treatment of a perforated duodenal ulcer?

Nothing by mouth (NPO), IV Fluids (IVF), antibiotics, and surgery

What is a life-threatening complication of a posterior duodenal ulcer?

Massive hemorrhage from erosion into the gastroduodenal artery

What are the key steps in the initial management of any patient with a severe upper GI bleed?

ABCs, IV fluids (via bilateral large peripheral IVs), nasogastric tube (NGT) suction, gastric lavage, blood transfusion if necessary

What is the most important diagnostic imaging test in a patient with a severe upper GI bleed?

Endoscopy

What type of treatment can be administered during endoscopy in a patient with an upper GI bleed?

Injection of bleeding vessel with sclerosing or vasoconstrictive agents

What type of treatment is indicated in patients with GI bleeding refractory to endoscopic treatment?

Surgery

What is the differential diagnosis of an upper GI bleed?

Duodenal ulcer (40%), gastric ulcer (10–20%), gastritis (15–20%), varices (10%), Mallory-Weiss tear (10%)

What term is used to describe a small esophageal tear near the GE junction, commonly occurring after retching, that may cause minor self-limited upper GI bleeding?

Mallory-Weiss tear

What cause of upper GI bleeding has the highest potential for rapid, life-threatening exsanguination?

Esophageal varices

Name the type of ulcer defined below:

Acute gastric ulcer found in burn and trauma victims

Curling's ulcer

Acute gastric ulcer associated with head trauma or surgery causing elevated intracranial pressure

Cushing's ulcer

Ulcer at a GI anastomotic site

Marginal ulcer

Name the type of gastritis associated with the following findings:

Autoimmune disorder with Autoantibodies to parietal cells and IF, Achlorhydria, pernicious Anemia, and Aging

Type A (fundal) chronic gastritis (remember the five As for Type A)

"Coffee-ground emesis" from mucosal inflammation

Acute (stress) gastritis

H. pylori infection

Type B (antral) chronic gastritis (B = bug)

NSAID ingestion

Type B (antral) chronic gastritis

Increased risk of PUD and gastric carcinoma

Type B (antral) chronic gastritis

Critically ill patients

Acute (stress) gastritis

What percentage of gastric tumors are malignant?

90–95% (95% are carcinomas)

What are the common presenting symptoms in a patient with gastric carcinoma?

Pain, anorexia, and weight loss

What are the major risk factors for gastric carcinoma?

Age >60, diets rich in nitrates, and chronic gastritis

What histopathologic finding in gastric cancer is associated with prognosis?

Depth of invasion

What is the diagnostic test of choice in a patient with suspected gastric carcinoma?

EGD with biopsies and endoscopic ultrasound to determine depth of invasion and nodal metastases

What are the three main patterns of gastric tumor growth?	Ulcerating (most common), fungating, and diffusely infiltrating (linitis plastica)
Provide the term associated with each of the following statements:	
Metastases to the pouch of Douglas in the pelvis	Blumer's shelf
Metastases to the ovary	Krukenberg tumor
Metastases to the left supraclavicular fossa	Virchow's node
Periumbilical lymph node metastases	Sister Mary Joseph's node

Gallbladder

What are the risk factors for cholelithiasis?	**Four Fs**: Fertile, Fat, Forty years old, and Female
What is the typical presentation of cholelithiasis?	Postprandial right upper quadrant (RUQ) pain (usually after fatty meals) with N/V
What are the two types of stones found in the gall bladder?	Cholesterol (75%) and pigment stones (25%)
Name the type of gallstone associated with each of the following:	
Native American	Cholesterol stone
Congenital hemoglobinopathy, hemolytic anemia	Pigment stone
Radiopaque	Pigment stone
Crohn's disease, cystic fibrosis	Cholesterol stone
Rapid weight loss (i.e., after gastric bypass)	Cholesterol stone
What is the diagnostic test for cholelithiasis?	RUQ ultrasound (98% sensitive and specific!)
What are five possible complications of cholelithiasis?	1. Acute cholecystitis 2. Choledocholithiasis 3. Gallstone pancreatitis 4. Gallstone ileus 5. Cholangitis
What is the treatment for symptomatic cholelithiasis?	Elective cholecystectomy

What are the indications for surgery in an asymptomatic patient?	Sickle cell disease and porcelain gallbladder ($\uparrow$ risk of CA)
What term is used to describe prolonged blockage of the cystic duct by an impacted stone leading to inflammation, infection, and possible gangrene of the gallbladder?	Acute cholecystitis
How does the pain differ in cholecystitis compared to cholelithiasis?	Pain in cholecystitis is more severe and prolonged
What physical examination finding is characterized by inspiratory arrest upon deep palpation of the RUQ in cholecystitis?	Murphy's sign (acute cholecystitis)
What are the other common signs and symptoms of cholecystitis?	Fever, N/V, tender gallbladder, leukocytosis, and referred right subscapular pain
What are three common findings on U/S in a patient with acute cholecystitis?	1. Gallbladder wall thickning 2. Pericholecystic fluid 3. Pressure of stones
What test may be done in a patient with acute cholecystitis when the ultrasound (U/S) is equivocal?	Hepatobiliary iminodiacetic acid (HIDA) scan (failure to visualize the gallbladder $\rightarrow$ acute cholecystitis)
What is the treatment of acute cholecystitis?	IVF, antibiotics, and early (<72 h) or late (6 weeks) cholecystectomy
Define choledocholithiasis.	Presence of gallstones within the common bile duct
What is the treatment for choledocholithiasis?	1. Endoscopic retrograde cholangiopancreatography (ERCP) with papillotomy and stone removal 2. Common bile duct exploration
What are two common complications of choledocholithiasis?	Cholangitis and pancreatitis
What is cholangitis?	Infection of the biliary tree 2° to obstruction
What are the two most common causes of bile duct obstruction?	Gallstones and malignancy
Name five classic signs and symptoms of obstructive jaundice.	1. Jaundice 2. Pruritus 3. Dark urine 4. Clay-colored stool 5. Weight loss (chronic)

What is Charcot's triad of cholangitis?	RUQ pain, jaundice, and fever/chills
What is Reynold's pentad of cholangitis?	Charcot's triad + shock and altered mental status
What is Courvoisier's sign?	Painless enlargement of the gallbladder with jaundice caused by carcinoma of the head of the pancreas
What are the common lab abnormalities in a patient with cholangitis?	Leukocytosis, ↑ direct bilirubin, and ↑ alkaline phosphatase (sensitive for bile duct inflammation)
What is the diagnostic gold standard for cholangitis?	ERCP
What organism most commonly causes cholangitis?	*Escherichia coli*
What is the treatment for cholangitis?	IVF, antibiotics, and relief of obstruction (ERCP with papillotomy, percutaneous transhepatic cholangiography [PTC] with catheter placement, or surgery)
Name two important complications of chronic cholangitis.	Cholangiocarcinoma and cirrhosis
What is the common comorbidity in patients with sclerosing cholangitis?	Inflammatory bowel disease (60%)
What is the surgical treatment of sclerosing cholangitis?	Removal of extrahepatic bile ducts (due to ↑ CA risk) and hepatoenteric anastomosis or transplant procedure
What is the most common type of gallbladder malignancy?	Adenocarcinoma (90%)
What are the major risk factors for gallbladder cancer?	Gallstones and porcelain gallbladder (10% have CA)
What is the name for malignancy of the intra- or extrahepatic bile ducts?	Cholangiocarcinoma
What are the major risk factors for cholangiocarcinoma?	Ulcerative colitis, sclerosing cholangitis, and thorotrast contrast dye
What is the name of a tumor at the junction of the left and right hepatic ducts?	Klatskin tumor
What surgery is typically performed for a distal cholangiocarcinoma?	Whipple procedure (pancreatico-duodenectomy)

Pancreas

Name nine causes of acute pancreatitis.	"GET SMASHeD" Gallstones Ethanol, ERCP Trauma Steroids Mumps (viruses) Autoimmune disorder Scorpion sting Hyperlipidemia Drugs (especially didanosine [DDI])
What term is used to refer to periumbilical and flank ecchymosis in hemorrhagic pancreatitis?	Cullen's sign and Grey-Turner sign (respectively)
Name six complications of acute pancreatitis.	1. Systemic inflammatory response syndrome (SIRS) 2. Necrosis 3. Psuedocyst formation 4. Pancreatic ascites 5. Fistula formation 6. GI or biliary obstruction
What are two classic radiologic findings on abdominal x-ray (AXR) in acute pancreatitis?	1. A **sentinel loop** of dilated bowel in left upper quadrant (LUQ) next to inflamed pancreas 2. The **colon cutoff sign**: Distended transverse colon with an absence of colonic gas distal to the splenic flexure
What is the most appropriate radiologic study for severe pancreatitis?	Abdominal computed tomography (CT)
What other test should be included in the diagnostic W/U of suspected gallstone pancreatitis?	RUQ ultrasound (to look for gallstones)
How many days after a bout of gallstone pancreatitis should a cholecystectomy be performed?	3–5 days after resolution of pancreatitis
In a patient undergoing cholecystectomy for a history of (h/o) gallstone pancreatitis, what test should be done intraoperatively?	Intraoperative cholangiogram (to rule out choledocholithiasis)
How is prognosis estimated in a patient with acute pancreatitis?	Ranson's criteria: 0–2 positives (<5% mortality rate), 3–4 (15%), 5–6 (40%), 7–8 (~100%)

What are the Ranson's criteria at presentation?	1. Age >55 2. WBC >16,000 3. Glucose >200 mg/dL 4. AST >250 5. LDH >350
What are the Ranson's criteria after 48 h?	1. Base deficit >4 2. ↑ in (BUN) >5 3. Fluid sequestration >6 L 4. Ca^{2+} <8.5 5. ↓ In Hct >10% 6. PaO_2 <60
Name four common laboratory abnormalities in acute pancreatitis.	1. ↑↑ Serum amylase (within 24 h) 2. ↑↑ Serum lipase (72–96 h) 3. Hypocalcemia 4. Glycosuria
What is the difference between a true cyst and a pseudocyst?	A true cyst is lined by epithelial cells; a pseudocyst is lined by fibrous tissue
When should a pseudocyst be drained interventionally?	If the cyst is greater than 6 cm for 6 weeks (50% resolve spontaneously), or if it is infected
What are the procedures for interval pseudocyst drainage?	Cystogastrostomy, cystojejunostomy, and cystoduodenostomy
Name five common causes of chronic pancreatitis.	**ABCCD** **A**lcoholism (#1 in adults) **B**iliary tract disease **C**ystic fibrosis (#1 in kids) **C**a^{2+} (hypercalcemia) **D**ivisum (pancreas divisum)
What is a classic diagnostic finding seen on AXR in chronic pancreatitis?	Calcification of the pancreas
What are two clinical signs of pancreatic insufficiency?	Diabetes (inadequate endocrine function) and steatorrhea (inadequate exocrine function)
What is the greatest risk factor for pancreatic cancer?	Smoking (↑ risk threefold)
Most pancreatic tumors are found in what region of the pancreas?	Two-thirds of pancreatic tumors are found in the pancreatic head

What is a common clinical consequence of a mass in the pancreatic head?	Obstructive, painless jaundice causing malabsorption and Courvoisier's (enlarged, palpable) gallbladder
What is Trousseau's *syndrome*?	Migratory superficial thrombophlebitis associated with visceral cancer, commonly pancreatic adenocarcinoma
What are two serologic markers of pancreatic cancer?	Carcinoembryonic antigen (CEA) and CA 19–9
What is the prognosis for pancreatic adenocarcinoma?	4% 5-year survival
What surgical procedure is commonly used for resection of a tumor in the head of the pancreas?	Whipple procedure (pancreatico-duodenectomy)
What characteristics of a tumor are contraindications for aggressive surgical intervention?	Vascular encasement, liver metastasis, peritoneal implants, distal lymph node metastasis, and distant metastasis

Liver

Name the most common…	
Benign liver tumor	Hemangioma
Primary liver cancer	Hepatocellular carcinoma (hepatoma)
Liver cancer	Metastasis
What is the feared complication of a hepatic hemangioma?	Hemorrhage (do NOT biopsy)
What is the treatment of a hepatic hemangioma?	Observation (surgery only if symptomatic)
What liver tumor is associated with oral contraceptives and anabolic steroids?	Hepatic adenoma
What is the treatment of a hepatic adenoma?	Discontinue birth control pills and observation
Name the two main types of liver abscesses.	Pyogenic and parasitic
What pathogen most frequently causes parasitic abscesses?	*Entamoeba histolytica*

What are the symptoms of a parasitic abscess caused by E. *histolytica*?	RUQ pain, fever, and bloody diarrhea
What is the treatment of a parasitic abscess?	IV metronidazole (surgery only if refractory)
What diagnosis is suggested by the presence of multiple small hepatic cysts on CT scan?	Infection with Echinococcus (eosinophilia and a $\oplus$ heme agglutination test are also common)
What procedure is contraindicated in treatment of echinococcal cysts?	Aspiration (requires open procedure to avoid contamination of peritoneal cavity)
Name the three most common organisms found in a pyogenic liver abscess.	*E. coli*, *Klebsiella*, and *Proteus*

Name the major risk factors for hepatocellular carcinoma.

"WATCH for **ABC"**

Wilson's disease

α-1-**A**ntitrypsin

Carcinogens (e.g., aflatoxin B_1, polyvinyl chloride)

Hemochromatosis

Alcoholic cirrhosis

Hepatitis **B**

Hepatitis **C**

Where is the most common site of metastasis for hepatocellular carcinoma?	Lung
What are the treatment options for hepatocellular carcinoma?	Surgical resection, chemoembolization, local ablation, or transplantation (monitor with α-fetoprotein)

Spleen

What are the indications for splenectomy in a patient with idiopathic thrombocytopenic purpura?	Failed corticosteroid treatment
Name three absolute indications for splenectomy.	1. Hereditary spherocytosis 2. Splenic tumors 3. **Massive** splenic trauma or spontaneous rupture
What is the main postsplenectomy complication?	Overwhelming postsplenectomy sepsis (OPSS)

What are the three main organisms responsible for OPSS?	*Streptococcus pneumoniae, Neisseria meningitidis,* and *Haemophilus influenzae* (all are **encapsulated**)
What are commonly administered to prevent OPSS?	Vaccinations

Hernias

Name the two factors that contribute to hernia formation.	Increased abdominal pressure (heavy lifting, cough, straining, pregnancy, ascites, obesity) and congenital defects

Name the hernia descriptor
defined below:

Hernia sac that can be reduced into normal anatomic location	Reducible
Hernia sac that cannot be reduced	Incarcerated
Incarcerated hernia sac causing hernia contents to become ischemic and eventually necrotic	Strangulated (needs emergent surgery)

Name the type of hernia described
below:

Inguinal hernia that protrudes from the peritoneal cavity *lateral* to the epigastric vessels; results from a patent processus vaginalis	Indirect inguinal hernia
Inguinal hernia that protrudes from the peritoneal cavity *medial* to the epigastric vessels	Direct inguinal hernia (hernia usually passes through Hasselbach's triangle-weakness of transversalis fascia)
Hernia protruding through the femoral sheath in the femoral canal medial to the femoral vein	Femoral hernia
Hernia protruding through the esophageal hiatus	Hiatal hernia (commonly leads to acid reflux disease)
Incarcerated hernia involving only one side of the bowel wall	Richter's hernia
Most common hernia in both males and females	Indirect inguinal hernia
Hernia that is more common in females than males	Femoral hernia

Type of hernia that may result in gangrenous bowel without causing small bowel obstruction (SBO)	Richter's hernia
Name three common complications of a hernia.	Pain, SBO, and necrosis of strangulated bowel
What is the definitive treatment for a hernia?	Surgical repair

Small Intestine

What condition commonly presents with abdominal discomfort, N/V, distension, cramping, and high-pitched bowel sounds?	SBO
What are the two most common causes of SBO?	Adhesions and hernias
What are five less common causes of SBO?	1. Neoplasms 2. Intussusception 3. Volvulus 4. Gallstone ileus 5. Crohn's disease
What type of hernia needs to be ruled out on physical examination in a patient with suspected SBO?	Incarcerated hernia
What are the three common findings in a patient with strangulated bowel?	Leukocytosis, tachycardia, and peritoneal signs
What is the key component of the history in a patient with suspected SBO?	Previous abdominal surgery (leading to adhesions)
What is the initial management of an adhesive SBO?	NPO, IVF, and NGT suction
What radiographic studies are commonly performed in patients with suspected SBO?	Acute abdominal series (upright AP chest XR, upright abdominal XR, and flat-plate abdominal XR)
What are three common findings on AXR in a patient with SBO?	Distended loops of bowel, air-fluid levels, and paucity of gas in colon/rectum
Define partial SBO.	Incomplete bowel obstruction with the presence of colonic gas
What is the classic acid-base disturbance in SBO?	Hypovolemic hypochloremic hypokalemic alkalosis (secondary to vomiting or nasogastric suction)

Why do patients with SBO develop hypokalemia?	Alkalosis drives K^+ into cells
What finding on urinalysis is characteristic of SBO?	Paradoxical aciduria
Why does aciduria occur?	H^+ exchanged for Na^+ during fluid resuscitation
What is the treatment of a *partial* SBO?	Conservative management and close monitoring
What is the treatment for a *complete* SBO?	Surgery
What type of obstruction is commonly associated with cramping abdominal pain, distention, nausea, and *feculent* vomitus?	Large bowel obstruction (LBO)
What are the three most common causes of LBO?	Colon CA, diverticulitis, and volvulus
What is the assumed cause of LBO until proven otherwise?	Colon cancer
What are the three studies necessary in the evaluation of LBO?	Contrast enema, CT scan, or colonoscopy if patient stable

Colon

What are the two most common causes of lower GI bleed (LGIB)?	Diverticulosis and angiodysplasia (arteriovenous malformation)
Which of the two most common etiologies for LGIB is most likely to present with intermittent bleeding?	Angiodysplasia
What is the source of bleeding in diverticular disease?	Erosion of a diverticulum into a colonic blood vessel
In what age group is diverticular disease most common?	>60 years old
What is the most common presenting symptom of diverticulitis?	Left lower quadrant (LLQ) pain
What the strongest risk factor for diverticular disease?	Low-fiber diet
Name the best radiologic test for the diagnosis of acute diverticulitis.	Abdominal/pelvic CT
What is the most common site of diverticular disease?	Sigmoid colon (95%)

Name four common complications of diverticulitis.	1. Abscess 2. Peritonitis 3. Fistula formation 4. Obstruction
Patients status post (s/p) hysterectomy are at increased risk of developing what complication of diverticulitis?	Enterovaginal fistula
What is the treatment of an initial attack of diverticulitis?	NPO, IVF, and antibiotics (ABX) (enteric and anaerobic coverage)
What is the risk of recurrence of an attack of diverticulitis after an initial episode?	33%
When is elective surgery indicated for diverticulitis?	After the second attack or after the first attack in a young, diabetic, or immunosuppressed patient
What must be ruled out in *every* patient with diverticulitis?	Colorectal cancer
What is volvulus and where does it most commonly occur?	Complete twisting of the bowel around its mesenteric base occurring most commonly in the sigmoid colon in elderly patients
How is volvulus diagnosed?	Sigmoidoscopy (also therapeutic for a nonstrangulated volvulus) or contrast enema
What inflammatory disease is often caused by overgrowth of exotoxin-producing bacteria?	Pseudomembranous colitis
What organism is most commonly responsible for pseudomembranous colitis?	*Clostridium difficile*
What tests are used for the diagnosis of pseudomembranous colitis?	Colonoscopy revealing pseudomembranes or *C. difficile* toxin detected in stool
What is the *early* finding in acute mesenteric ischemia?	Abdominal pain out of proportion to examination
What are the *late* findings in acute mesenteric ischemia?	Bloody diarrhea, fever, and peritonitis (80% mortality)
List the three main causes of mesenteric ischemia.	Embolization (atrial fibrillation), thrombosis (atherosclerotic plaque), or nonocclusive ischemia ($\downarrow$ CO or medications)

What is the drug classically associated with mesenteric ischemia?	Digoxin
What is the triad of symptoms in chronic mesenteric ischemia?	Postprandial abdominal pain, weight loss, and food aversion/fear
How many vessels must be occluded to produce symptomatic chronic mesenteric ischemia?	Two out of three mesenteric arteries (celiac, superior mesenteric artery [SMA], inferior mesenteric artery [IMA])
Ischemic bowel disease commonly affects which part of the GI tract?	"Watershed" areas (splenic flexure, rectosigmoid junction)
What is the diagnostic test of choice for mesenteric ischemia?	Arteriogram

Name the autosomal dominant syndrome associated with each of the following findings:

Colonic polyps, osteomas, and soft tissue tumors; associated with abnormal dentition	Gardner's syndrome
Hundreds of colonic polyps; malignant potential ~100%	Familial adenomatous polyposis (FAP)
Colonic polyps and central nervous system (CNS) tumors; malignant potential ~100%	Turcot's syndrome
Defect in DNA repair → many colonic lesions (especially proximal); malignant potential ~50%	Hereditary nonpolyposis colorectal carcinoma (HNPCC) or Lynch's syndrome
Benign, hamartomas of GI tract; melanotic pigmentation of hand, mouth, and genitalia; no malignant potential (but ↑ risk of other tumors)	Peutz-Jeghers syndrome

Name the type of neoplastic polyp:

Usually benign and pedunculated; most common type	Tubular adenoma (75%)
Highly malignant; sessile tumor with fingerlike projections	Villous adenoma
Shares features of both other types of polyps	Tubulovillous adenoma
Name five major risk factors for colon cancer.	1. Colonic villous adenomas 2. Inflammatory bowel disease 3. ↓ Fiber, ↑ animal fat diet 4. Age (>50) 5. Positive family/personal history

How does colorectal carcinoma typically present?	Left side lesion → constipation; right side lesion → anemia (from occult blood loss)
In an older adult male with iron-deficiency anemia what diagnosis must be ruled out?	Colon cancer (second most common cancer in the United States)
What is the current recommendation for colon cancer screening?	Hemoccult and digital rectal examination (DRE) every year >50 y/o Flexible sigmoidoscopy every 3–5 years >50 y/o, *or* colonoscopy every 10 years **Note:** If +family history (⊕ FH), start screening 10 years before age of family member with CA at diagnosis
What is the gold standard for the diagnosis of colon cancer?	Colonoscopy with tissue biopsy
How does rectal CA usually present?	Hematochezia, tenesmus, and incomplete evacuation of stool
What is the primary therapy for colorectal cancer?	Surgical resection (adjuvant therapy for Stage III)
What marker can be used to follow progression of colon cancer treatment?	CEA. **Note:** CEA is not specific enough to serve as an adequate screening method

Appendix

What are the two most common causes of appendiceal obstruction?	Obstruction of the appendix due to fecalith and lymphoid hyperplasia
What is the classic presentation of appendicitis?	Onset of periumbilical pain (referred pain) followed by N/V, *anorexia* and later, right lower quadrant (RLQ) pain (due to localized peritoneal irritation)
In what order do patients with appendicitis typically experience the symptoms of abdominal pain and N/V?	Pain precedes N/V in appendicitis; **Note:** Nausea and vomiting followed by abdominal pain suggests gastroenteritis
How is the diagnosis of appendicitis made?	By history and physical examination

What are the classic physical examination findings in a patient with appendicitis?	Low-grade fever, RLQ pain with local signs of peritoneal irritation (guarding, rebound tenderness)
What lab tests are typically ordered in the W/U of appendicitis?	CBC (leukocytosis), urinalysis (r/o UTI or calculus), and β–hCG (**all** female patients)
What radiologic test can be done when the diagnosis of appendicitis is in doubt?	Abdominal/pelvic CT
What radiologic test is best to evaluate ovarian causes of lower abdominal pain?	Ultrasound
What is the most common emergency abdominal surgery performed in the United States?	Appendectomy
Name each physical examination finding described below:	
Point of maximal tenderness one-third from the anterior iliac spine to the umbilicus	McBurney's point
Pain in RLQ on palpation of LLQ	Rovsing's sign
Pain on internal rotation of the leg with both hip and knee flexed	Obturator sign
Pain on extension of hip with knee in full flexion	Psoas sign
What is the treatment of appendicitis?	IVF, antibiotics, and surgery
What are two common feared complications of ruptured appendicitis?	Peritonitis and abscess formation
How is an abscess caused by appendicitis managed?	Percutaneous drainage, antibiotics, and interval appendectomy 6–8 weeks later
How long should a patient with appendicitis be treated with antibiotics?	24 h (nonperforated), 7–10 days (perforated)
What is the most common tumor of the appendix?	Carcinoid tumor
What type of cells give rise to carcinoid tumors?	Neuroendocrine (Kulchitcky) cells
What substances are secreted from carcinoid tumors?	Serotonin, histamine, and prostaglandins

What type of carcinoid tumors tend to be the most aggressive?	Ileal, gastric, and colonic
Name five clinical findings of carcinoid syndrome.	1. Vasomotor dysfunction 2. GI hypermotility 3. Bronchoconstriction 4. Hepatomegaly 5. Right-sided heart valve degeneration
Metastasis of a carcinoid tumor to what organ may result in carcinoid syndrome?	Liver
What lab test is used to diagnose carcinoid syndrome?	5-hydroxyindoleacetic acid (5-HIAA) in urine
What is the treatment for a carcinoid tumor?	Surgical resection (octreotide for carcinoid syndrome)

Breast

What is the second leading cause of cancer death among women?	Breast cancer
Name five risk factors for breast cancer.	1. Age 2. FH of premenopausal breast cancer 3. Nulliparity 4. Age of menarche (<13)/age at menopause (>55) 5. First pregnancy after 34
Name five conditions that increase the risk of developing breast cancer.	1. Lobular/ductal carcinoma in situ (LCIS/DCIS) 2. Atypical hyperplasia 3. BRCA I/II gene positive 4. Sclerosing adenitis 5. Cancer in contralateral breast
What is the most common site of breast cancer?	Upper outer breast quadrant
What are the classic signs and symptoms of breast cancer?	Mass, dimple, nipple retraction, nipple discharge, rash, local edema, and enlarged axillary lymph nodes
Name two imaging tools used to detect breast cancer.	1. Mammography 2. Ultrasound (best for women <30 y/o with fibrous breast tissue)
What findings on mammography are suspicious for malignancy?	Stellate or spiculated mass and microcalcifications

What is the diagnostic evaluation of a nonpalpable, suspicious lesion on mammography?	Stereotactic or needle localized excisional biopsy

Name the breast disease associated with the following statements:

Most common breast malignancy	Ductal carcinoma (90%)
Most common tumor in young women	Fibroadenoma (benign)
Peau d'orange (edema of the dermis) appearance	Inflammatory carcinoma
Most common cause of bloody nipple discharge	Intraductal papilloma
Tumor cells invade epidermal layer of skin near the nipple	Paget's disease of breast
Increased risk of CA in *same* breast	DCIS (premalignant)
Increased risk of CA in *either* breast	LCIS (premalignant)
Solid, mobile, and well-circumscribed round breast mass	Fibroadenoma (benign)
Breast tenderness with menstrual cycle; cysts and nodules	Fibrocystic disease (benign)
Superficial infection of breast; usually caused by *Staphylococcus aureus;* associated with breast feeding	Mastitis

Name the treatment for each of the following breast diseases:

Fibroadenoma	Observation ± biopsy
Fibrocystic disease	Vitamin E and NSAIDs (if cysts present—aspiration; if bloody aspirate, then biopsy)
Mastitis	Continue breast feeding; antibiotics
DCIS	Lumpectomy plus x-ray therapy (XRT) or total simple mastectomy
LCIS	Close follow-up (f/u) or *bilateral* simple mastectomy in high-risk patients
Invasive carcinoma	Lumpectomy plus x-ray XRT or modified radical mastectomy (both ± chemotherapy); sentinel lymph node biopsy axillary lymph node dissection

Name two potential complications of modified radical mastectomy.	Arm lymphedema and injury to nerves
What are the major side effects of tamoxifen?	Endometrial cancer and deep venous thrombosis (DVT)
What are the screening recommendations for breast cancer prevention?	1. Monthly self-breast examinations 2. Annual breast examinations by physician >40 y/o 3. Annual mammogram after age 50

VASCULAR

What are the two major risk factors for peripheral vascular disease (PVD)?	Smoking and diabetes mellitus (DM)
Name two common presenting symptoms of PVD.	Intermittent claudication and ischemic rest pain
What are the signs of PVD?	Absent pulses, trophic skin changes (shiny skin, loss of hair, thickened toenails), dependent rubor, muscular atrophy, and necrotic tissue (gangrene)
On examination, how can one differentiate between a foot ulcer caused by ischemia versus venous stasis?	Ischemic foot ulcers commonly occur on the toes or feet; ulcers due to stasis commonly occur on the medial malleolus
What are the symptoms of claudication?	Reproducible pain in the lower extremities (usually calf muscles) exacerbated by walking and relieved by rest
Is claudication limb-threatening?	No (only 5% will lose limb in 5 years)
Define ischemic rest pain.	Severe foot pain at rest, usually in the distal foot and arch, caused by PVD
What simple maneuver may bring some relief to patients with ischemic rest pain?	Placing foot in dependent position (e.g., over side of bed)
What does ischemic rest pain signify?	Limb-threatening condition (85% of patients will lose the affected limb in 5 years)
What is the triad of impotence, buttock claudication, and gluteus muscle atrophy called?	Leriche's syndrome (caused by aortailiac occlusive disease)

What is the gold standard for the diagnosis of PVD?

Arteriogram (always needed preoperatively)

What conservative measures are commonly taken in the management of a patient with PVD?

Smoking cessation, exercise, and aspirin ± clopidogrel

What are the interventional treatment options for PVD?

1. Percutaneous transluminal angioplasty (PTA)—best for focal, short disease of proximal vessels
2. Surgical revascularization
3. Amputation

What are the surgical indications for PVD?

Rest pain, tissue loss, and incapacitating claudication

What are the "six Ps" of acute arterial occlusion?

Pain, Pallor, Pulselessness, Paralysis, Poikilothermia, and Parasthesias

What is the most common cause of acute arterial occlusion?

Embolization (85% are caused by thrombi formed in the heart)

What are the treatment options for acute arterial occlusion?

1. Surgical embolectomy
2. Surgical bypass
3. Thrombolytic therapy

What medication must be started in every patient with suspected arterial occlusion?

Heparin

What are the signs and symptoms of compartment syndrome?

Reperfusion injury causing calf pain (especially on passive stretch), tenderness, paralysis, and parasthesias. **Note:** Pulses may still be present in affected compartment.

What is the definitive treatment for compartment syndrome?

Emergent fasciotomy

Name five risk factors for development of an Abdominal aortic aneurysm (AAA).

Atherosclerosis, smoking, hypertension, age (>60), and gender (M:F-4:1)

Where is the most common site of an AAA?

Infrarenal

State the risk of rupture annually of an AAA with each of the following diameters:

<5cm

4% (9% in 5 years)

Between 5 and 7 cm

7% (35% in 5 years)

>7 cm

20% (75% in 5 years)

What are the indications for surgery in a patient with an AAA?

AAA >5 cm or growth >4 mm/year or if symptomatic

What is the classic clinical triad of a ruptured AAA?	Abdominal pain, hypotension, and pulsatile abdominal mass
What is the treatment for a ruptured AAA?	Emergent operation (50% surgical mortality rate)
What are the common postoperative complications in a patient after an AAA repair?	MI (#1 cause of postoperative death), colonic ischemia, anterior spinal syndrome (caused by occlusion of the artery of Adamkiewicz), or acute renal failure

ORTHOPEDICS

For each description, name the associated orthopedic injury and its treatment:

Fx of the fifth metacarpal resulting from closed fist striking a hard object	Boxer Fx—closed reduction (CR) and ulnar splint (pinning for excess angulation); **Note:** If skin is broken → debride and ABX for presumed human oral pathogen infection
Most commonly fractured carpal bone → tenderness in anatomical snuffbox	Scaphoid Fx—thumb spica cast. **Note:** Radiographs may be normal up to 2 weeks; ↑ risk for avascular necrosis (AVN) and nonunion
Most common Fx of wrist; fall on outstretched hand (FOOSH) → Fx of distal radius with dorsal displacement of distal fragment	Colles' Fx—CR and cast immobilization
Ulnar diaphyseal Fx and dislocation of radial head	Monteggia Fx (aka "nightstick Fx")—CR of radial head and open reduction, internal fixation (ORIF) of ulna
Radial head subluxation; occurs after being forcefully pulled by the hand	Nursemaid elbow—manual reduction (supinate at 90° elbow flexion)
Radial nerve palsy resulting from direct trauma to upper arm	Humerus Fx—hanging arm cast; functional bracing
Radial shaft Fx with dislocation of distal radioulnar joint	Galeazzi Fx—ORIF and casting of arm in supination
Most common shoulder dislocation (95%); due to subcoracoid dislocation	Anterior shoulder dislocation—CR, sling (2–6 weeks), intense rehabilitation
Most common Fx in school-age children; may threaten the brachial artery	Supracondylar Fx of humerus—CR and percutaneous pinning; **Note:** ↑ risk of Volkmann's ischemic contracture of forearm

Most frequently fractured long bone in kids; sometimes related to birth trauma	Clavicular Fx (commonly middle third)—sling
Pain/tenderness over anterior humeral head resulting from impingement; ⊕ Neer's sign	Rotator cuff injury—NSAIDs; steroid injection; surgery if refractory to steroids
Most common type of hip dislocation; severe trauma (*dashboard injury*) → internally rotated, flexed, and adducted hip	Posterior hip dislocation—**orthopedic emergency**: reduction under sedation; f/u with serial imaging for 2 years (↑ risk of AVN)
Fx associated with falls in osteoporotic women and ↑ risk of AVN and DVT; results in shortened, externally rotated leg	Femoral neck Fx—ORIF and parallel pinning or hemiarthroplasty; anticoagulate to ↓ risk of DVT
Fx most commonly associated with fat emboli syndrome (dyspnea, hypoxia,confusion, and scleral petechiae)	Fx of the femur—intramedullary nailing of femur
Lower extremity Fx after landing on foot from large vertical drop; part of "lover's triad" (with lumbar compression Fx and forearm Fx)	Calcaneal Fx—ORIF
Most common type of ankle sprain (90%); results from ankle plantar-flexion	Lateral sprain—**RICE: R**est, **I**ce, **C**ompression, **E**levation (to ↓ swelling)
Extreme inversion of the foot → Fx of fibula and avulsion at base of the fifth metatarsal	Jones' Fx—immobilization without weight bearing
Extreme eversion of the foot → Fx of fibula and avulsion of the medial malleolus	Pott's Fx—ORIF

ABDOMINAL PAIN

State the most common causes of abdominal pain in each of the following locations:

Right lower quadrant

1. Appendicitis
2. Gynecologic causes: ovarian cyst, PID, ectopic pregnancy, etc.
3. Inflammatory bowel disease-Crohn's disease >> UC
4. Meckel's diverticulitis
5. Intussusception

Left lower quadrant	1. Diverticulitis 2. Gynecologic causes (same as RLQ pain) 3. Obstructing mass 4. Constipation 5. Sigmoid volvulus (may be generalized)
Right upper quadrant	1. Cholecystitis 2. Choledocholithiasis/Cholethiasis 3. Cholangitis 4. Hepatitis 5. Hepatic tumor (commonly hepatoma) 6. R sided pneumonia
Epigastrium	1. Gastric or duodenal ulcer 2. Gastritis/gastroenteritis 3. Pancreatitis 4. MI **Note:** peritonitis, SBO, mesenteric ischemia, pneumonia, MI, gastroenteritis, may present with pain in any abdominal location

MAKE THE DIAGNOSIS

21 y/o male presents with hematemesis after ingestion of aspirin and seven shots of whiskey; PE: diaphoretic, ↑ HR, epigastric tenderness; EGD: edematous, friable reddened gastric mucosa	Acute gastritis
A patient with h/o PUD presents with melena; PE: ↑ HR, diaphoretic, epioastric abdominal pain; W/U: NGT aspirate is bloody; EGD: visible bleeding vessel distal to the pylorus	Bleeding duodenal ulcer
A patient with h/o multiple abdominal surgeries presents with crampy abdominal pain, N/V, and ↓ bowel movements; PE: hyperactive bowel sounds, abdominal distension; AXR: dilated small bowel loops, absent colonic gas, and multiple air-fluid levels	SBO

40 y/o obese, mother of four presents
with constant RUQ pain radiating to
right scapula, N/V; PE: fever, tenderness,
and respiratory pause induced by RUQ
palpation, painful palpable gallbladder;
W/U: ↑ WBC, ↑ ALP; U/S: thickened
gallbladder wall, pericholecystic fluid
with gallstones present

Acute cholecystitis

39 y/o male presents with dull, steady
epigastric pain radiating to the back
after an alcohol binge, N/V;
PE: fever, ↑ BP, epigastric tenderness,
gaurding, and distension; W/U: ↑↑
amylase/lipase, ↑ WBC; AXR:
sentinel loop, colon cutoff

Acute pancreatitis

65 y/o Black male with h/o smoking
presents with anorexia, weight loss,
pruritis, and painless jaundice;
PE: palpable nontender distended
gallbladder, migratory thrombophlebitis;
W/U: ↑ direct bilirubin, ALP, CEA, and
CA 19-9, Abdominal CT: mass in
head of pancreas

Pancreatic adenocarcinoma

60 y/o Black male with h/o GERD
presents with weight loss and
dysphagia; EGD: partially obstructing
mass near GE junction

Esophageal adenocarcinoma

61 y/o White female presents with
right-sided breast mass; PE: breast
dimpling, nipple retraction; W/U:
mammography shows irregular
speculated mass in upper outer
quadrant with calcifications

Breast cancer

24 y/o female presents with a
breast mass; PE: solid, mobile,
well-circumscribed rubbery breast
mass; W/U: U/S shows circumscribed,
homogeneous, oval-shaped,
hypoechoic mass

Fibroadenoma

65 y/o presents with severe worsening
LLQ pain, N/V, and diarrhea; PE: fever,
LLQ tenderness, local guarding and
rebound tenderness; W/U: ↑ WBC;
Abd CT: edematous colonic wall
with localized fluid collection

Diverticulitis

30 y/o female presents with periumbilical pain which has now migrated to the RLQ followed by anorexia, N/V; PE: low-grade fever, local RLQ guarding, rebound tenderness, RLQ tenderness upon LLQ palpation; W/U: β-hCG negative, $\uparrow$ WBC with left shift	Appendicitis
80 y/o White male smoker with h/o CAD presents with abrupt onset of severe abdominal and back pain; PE: $\downarrow$ BP, pulsatile abdominal mass	Abdominal aortic aneurysm
55 y/o presents with colicky abdominal pain, small-caliber stools, and occasional melena; PE: cachexia, abdominal discomfort, guaiac $\oplus$; W/U: colonoscopy shows obstructing mass seen in ascending colon	Right-sided colon carcinoma
80 y/o women presents with halitosis, dysphagia, and regurgitation of undigested foods; W/U: barium swallow shows posterior midline pouch greater than 2 cm in diameter arising just above the cricopharyngeus muscle	Zenker's diverticulum
55 y/o Asian female with h/o hepatitis B virus (HBV) presents with dull RUQ pain; PE: weight loss, painful hepatomegaly, ascites, jaundice; W/U: $\uparrow$ alanine transaminase/aspartate transaminase (ALT/AST), $\uparrow$ α-fetoprotein; Abd CT: mass seen in R lobe of liver	Hepatocellular carcinoma
55 y/o with h/o choledocholithiasis presents with fever, chills, and RUQ pain; PE: jaundice; W/U: $\uparrow$ WBC, bilirubin, and ALP; U/S: stone in common bile duct	Cholangitis
A patient presents to ED after motor vehicle accident (MVA) with LUQ abdominal pain and L shoulder tenderness; PE: guarding, rebound tenderness, $\downarrow$BP, $\uparrow$ HR; W/U: U/S: presence of intraabdominal fluid	Splenic laceration
43 y/o male presents with epigastric pain, diarrhea, and recurrent peptic ulcers; PE: epigastric tenderness; W/U: $\uparrow$ fasting gastrin levels, paradoxic $\uparrow$ in gastrin with secretin challenge; Octreotide scan: detect lesion in pancreas	Zollinger-Ellison syndrome

A trauma patient presents in the ED after MVA with right-sided pleuritic chest pain, dyspnea, and tachypnea; PE: ↓ BP, ⊕ JVD, unilateral absent of breath sounds and hyperresonance on R side, tracheal deviation away from R side

Tension pneumothorax

71 y/o with h/o atrial fibrillation presents with acute onset abdominal pain and bloody diarrhea; PE: writhing in pain, irregularly irregular heart rhythm, no peritoneal sign; W/U: arteriogram shows lack of visualization of the SMA and its branches

Acute mesenteric ischemia

72 y/o presents with recurrent, low-grade, painless hematochezia; PE: guaiac ⊕ stool; W/U: colonoscopy reveals slightly raised, discrete, scalloped lesion with visible draining vein in R colon

Angiodysplasia

73 y/o smoker with h/o atrial fibrillation and DM presents with acute onset of pain and numbness in L leg; PE: cool, pulseless L leg; W/U: arteriogram reveals complete occlusion of common femoral artery

Acute arterial occlusion

63 y/o Japanese male with h/o atrophic gastritis presents with weight loss, indigestion, epigastric pain, and vomiting; PE: supraclavicular lymph node; WU: anemia, ⊕ fecal occult blood

Gastric carcinoma

48 y/o with chronic watery diarrhea, hot flashes, and facial redness; PE: shows II/VI right-sided ejection murmur; W/U: ↑ 5-HIAA in urine

Carcinoid syndrome

40 y/o presents with dysphagia, regurgitation, and weight loss; W/U: barium swallow demonstrates dilated esophagus with distal narrowing (*bird beak*)

Achalasia

16 y/o with strong FH of colorectal CA presents with rectal bleeding and abdominal pain; W/U: anemia; Flexible sigmoidoscopy: >100 adenomatous polyps visualized

Familial adenomatous polyposis (FAP)

## CHAPTER 3

Neuroscience

Headache

Name the type of headache (migraine, tension, cluster, or sinus) associated with the following features:

Aspirin, nonsteroidal anti-inflammatory drugs (NSAIDs), sumatriptans, ergot alkaloids, and opiates may be used as abortive therapy	Migraine
Associated with nausea/vomiting, photophobia, phonophobia	Migraine
β-Blockers, calcium channel blockers, ergots, antidepressants, and depakote are used for prophylaxis	Migraine
Classic symptoms include unilateral frontotemporal cephalgia with aura and visual symptoms (e.g., scintillating scotoma)	Migraine
Course is characterized by periods of multiple headaches of the same character alternating with symptom-free intervals	Cluster
Findings include ipsilateral tearing, conjunctival injection, Horner's syndrome, and rhinorrhea	Cluster
Headaches described as pulsatile or throbbing	Migraine
Headaches may be precipitated by hormonal factors (eg. OCPs or menses), emotional or metabolic stress	Migraine
History of allergies	Sinus
Localized tenderness over sinsuses	Sinus

Most common type of headache in adults	Tension
Pathophysiology may relate to the effect of serotonin on cephalic blood vessels	Migraine
Patients often have a family history (FH) of headaches	Migraine
Symptoms are often eradicated by 100% O_2 by facemask	Cluster
Unilateral boring periorbital headache worst in the temporo-orbital region	Cluster
Vise-like, tightening bilateral pain associated with photophobia, phonophobia, neck tightness	Tension

What are the seven red flags of a headache?

1. Sudden onset of severe headache
2. Headache beginning after straining, valsalva, sexual activity, or awakens patient from sleep
3. Headache that is persistent and worsening over a period of weeks or months
4. Headache associated with focal neurologic findings or a change in mental status
5. Headache associated with meningeal signs (including nuchal rigidity, Brudzinski's or Kernig's sign)
6. Headache associated with fever
7. Headache in an patient who has never experienced a headache before

Seizures

Name the type of seizure associated with the following clinical findings:

Brief lapses of consciousness with or without rapid eye blinking, slight head, and limb jerking in a child	Absence seizure
First line of therapy may include valproate, phenytoin, carbamazepine, phenobarbital, or newer agents (levetiracetam, oxcarbazepine, lamotrigine)	Tonic-clonic seizure

Sudden, brief muscle contractions; first line of therapy includes valproate and clonazepam	Myoclonic seizures
Commonly mistaken as daydreaming in a young child	Absence seizure
First line of therapy includes ethosuximide and valproate	Absence seizure
Loss of consciousness followed by loss of postural control, a tonic phase of muscle contraction, and clonic phase of limb jerking	Tonic-clonic seizure
Motor, sensory, visual, psychic, or autonomic phenomena with preserved level of consciousness	Simple partial seizure
Three hertz spike-and-wave pattern on EEG	Absence seizure
May be associated with cyanosis and urinary or fecal incontinence; ↑ serum prolactin during postictal period	Tonic-clonic seizure
Motor, sensory, visual, psychic, or autonomic phenomena with preserved level of consciousness	Simple partial seizure
Motor, sensory, visual, psychic, or autonomic phenomena with diminished level of consciousness and/or postictal confusion	Complex partial seizure
Seizure interferes with a single neurologic modality (motor, sensory, or autonomic function) but does not cause loss of consciousness	Simple partial seizure
Seizure commonly involves the temporal lobe	Complex partial seizure

Cerebral Vasculature

Describe the artery that has been occluded in each of the following stroke syndromes:

Paresis and sensory loss of contralateral lower extremity	Anterior cerebral artery (ACA)
Hemiparesis, contralateral hemisensory loss, homonymous hemianopsia, aphasia	Middle cerebral artery (MCA) supplying the dominant hemisphere

Altered mental status, memory deficits, hemisensory loss, homonymous hemianopsia with macular sparing	Posterior cerebral artery (PCA)
Amaurosis fugax	Ophthalmic artery
Vertigo, cranial nerve (CN) palsies, impaired level of consciousness, dysarthria	Basilar artery
Sensory neglect and apraxia	Partial occlusion of the MCA supplying the nondominant hemisphere
Urinary incontinence, suck and grasp reflexes	MCA or ACA supplying the frontal lobe
Wernicke's aphasia (fluent speech without meaning; poor comprehension and word repetition)	Dominant inferior MCA
Broca's aphasia (nonfluent speech with poor repetition and normal comprehension)	Superior dominant MCA
What is the most common source of emboli that result in stroke?	Carotid atheroma
Name the term used to describe the infarction of white matter commonly associated with hypertension, diabetes, and carotid atherosclerosis.	Lacunar infarction
Name the term used to describe the infarction of gray matter commonly associated with sustained hypotension.	Watershed infarction
Cerebral edema may cause dangerous elevations in intracranial pressure (ICP) how long after a stroke?	Two to five days
What interventions are available for lowering ICP?	1. Elevate the head of the bed 2. IV mannitol/diuretics 3. Hyperventilation 4. Sedation 5. Cerebrospinal fluid (CSF) drainage (ventriculostomy)
Name the term used to describe a neurologic deficit caused by ischemia that resolves within 24 h.	Transient ischemic attack (TIA)
What is the primary radiologic study necessary in the workup (W/U) of stroke?	Computed tomography (CT) scan of the head **without contrast**

What radiologic study may be useful in determining the etiology of an ischemic stoke?	Cerebral angiography
What radiologic study can provide useful information about the etiology of a stroke if angiography is contraindicated?	Magnetic resonance angiography
What oral medications have been shown to improve outcome in patients with acute ischemic stroke?	Aspirin, clopidigrel, ticlodipine, and Aggrenox
What type of therapy is indicated in a patient at risk for cardioembolic stroke?	Anticoagulation with heparin followed by coumadin
What medical intervention has been shown to improve outcome in embolic stroke patients when they are treated within 3 h?	Tissue plasminogen activator (tPA)
What surgical intervention is indicated for patients with carotid atherosclerosis causing >70% compromise of the carotid lumen?	Carotid endarterectomy
What primary preventative measures are recommended in a patient at risk for ischemic stroke?	Smoking cessation, antihypertensive therapy, glycemic control in diabetics, cholesterol lowering therapy

Intracranial Hemorrhage

Name the type of intracranial hemorrhage associated with the following features:

Associated with cerebral arteriovenous malformations	Subarachnoid and intraparenchymal hemorrhage
Commonly caused by ruptured berry aneurysm; classically presents as "the worst headache of my life"	Subarachnoid hemorrhage
Commonly presents with headache and lethargy in a patient with focal motor and sensory defects	Intraparenchymal hemorrhage
Hematoma following the contour of a cerebral hemisphere on CT; due to laceration of bridging cerebral veins	Subdural hematoma

Lens-shaped hematoma on CT scan; due to laceration of middle meningeal artery due to fracture of the temporal bone	Epidural hematoma
Lumbar puncture (LP) must be performed in a patient with suspected intracranial hemorrhage even if CT scan is negative	Subarachnoid hemorrhage
Lucid interval followed by rapid decline in mental status	Epidural hematoma
May present with meningeal signs, CN palsies, seizures, and focal neurologic signs; bloody or xanthrochromic CSF on LP	Subarachnoid hemorrhage (secondary to ruptured aneurysm)
Most common type of intracranial hemorrhage from trauma	Subdural hematoma (commonly seen in alcoholics and the elderly)
Treated with emergent neurosurgical evacuation	Epidural hematoma (and subdural hematoma >1 cm or with midline shift)
Type of intracranial hemorrhage seen in patients with long-standing, poorly controlled hypertension	Intraparenchymal hemorrhage
What is the central principle in the management of hemorrhagic stroke?	Management of ICP (see above)
What is the fastest nonsurgical method for lowering ICP?	Hyperventilation

Brain Tumors

What are the most common types of intracranial tumors?	Metastatic tumors
Name the primary brain tumor associated with each of the following clinical or pathologic findings:	
Five-year survival of less than 4–5%	Glioblastoma multiforme (GBM)
Benign tumor derived form arachnoid cap cells with well-delineated margins	Meningioma
EBV ⊕ B-cell tumor of the CNS in AIDS patients	CNS lymphoma

Malignant pediatric tumor found exclusively in the posterior fossa	Medulloblastoma (metastasizes through CSF pathways)
Most common pediatric intracranial tumor	Juvenile pilocytic astrocytoma
Most common pediatric supratentorial tumor	Craniopharyngioma
Most common pituitary adenoma	Prolactinoma
Most common pituitary tumor	Pituitary adenoma
Most common primary brain tumor	Glioblastoma multiforme
Multiple lesions at presentation	CNS lymphoma
Small round blue cell tumor	Medulloblastoma
Tumor arising from ependymal lining of ventricular system	Ependymoma
Tumor characterized by highly malignant cells bordering necrotic areas	Glioblastoma multiforme
Tumor derived from Rathke's pouch	Craniopharyngioma
Tumor of the dorsal root that may grow in a dumbbell configuration through a vertebral foramen	Schwannoma
Tumor which originates from the vestibular division of CN VIII	Schwannoma
Two tumors often presenting with bitemporal hemianopia	Pituitary adenoma and craniopharyngioma
Type of tumor that may be found bilaterally in patients with neurofibromatosis II	Acoustic neuroma/Schwannoma
Vascular tumor of cerebellum and retina in patients with von Hippel-Lindau syndrome	Hemangioblastoma
What are the three modalities used in the treatment of a brain tumor?	1. Surgery 2. Chemotherapy 3. Radiation therapy

CNS Infections

What are the common symptoms of meningitis?	Fever, headache, neck stiffness, photophobia, change in mental status
What are the classic signs of meningitis?	Change in mental status and meningeal signs: Kernig's sign, Brudzinski's sign, and nuchal rigidity

What test is necessary to make the diagnosis of meningitis?	CSF analysis (usually obtained by LP)

Name the type of meningitis associated with the following CSF findings:

>1000 Polymorphonuclear leukocytes, ↓ glucose, ↑ protein	Bacterial meningitis
Increased lymphocytes, minor elevation in protein, normal CSF pressure	Viral meningitis
Increased lymphocytes, minor elevation in protein, dramatically ↓ glucose, elevated CSF pressure	Fungal meningitis
Increased lymphocytes, ↑ protein, ↓ glucose	TB meningitis

Name the most common bacterial pathogens responsible for causing meningitis and the appropriate treatment for each of the demographic groups:

<1 month	Group B strep (commonly *Streptococcus agalactiae*), *Escherichia coli, Listeria*
	Empiric treatment: Second generation cephalosporin and ampicillin; **Note:** There are other acceptable empiric antibiotic regimens
1–3 months	*Streptococcus pneumoniae, Neisseria meningitidis, Haemophilus influenzae* (less common today due to vaccinations)
	Empiric treatment: Second generation cephalosporin, vancomycin, and steroids
3 months—adulthood	*S. pneumoniae* (most common cause of meningitis in adults), *N. meningitidis*
	Treatment: Third generation cephalosporin, vancomycin and steroids
Associated with surgery or trauma to the CNS	*Staphylococcus aureus*
	Treatment: Vancomycin and ceftazidime

Adults >60 with chronic illness (including alcoholics)	*S. pneumoniae,* gram-negative bacilli, *Listeria*
	Treatment: Third generation cephalosporin, ampicillin, and steroids

Name seven complications of meningitis:

1. Hyponatremia
2. Seizures
3. Subdural effusion (especially with *H. influenzae* meningitis)
4. Cerebral edema
5. Subdural empyema
6. Brain abscess
7. Ventriculitis

Name the type of meningitis or encephalitis classically associated with the following features:

Argyll-Robertson pupil	Syphilis
Frequent cause of encephalitis and intracranial mass lesions in AIDS patients with CD4 count <200	Toxoplasmosis
Latin American immigrant with seizures	Neurocysticercosis (due to *Taenia solium*)
Lymphocytic meningitis, cranial neuropathy, and erythema chronicum migrans	Lyme disease
Maternal exposure to cat feces	Toxoplasmosis
Most common cause of viral encephalitis	Herpes simplex encephalitis
Most common type of fungal meningitis; commonly seen in immunosuppressed patients; birds are the host for the pathogen	Cryptococcal meningitis
Paresis and tabes dorsalis (sensory ataxia)	Syphilis
Ring-enhancing lesions associated with focal neurologic deficits	Toxoplasmosis
Subacute onset of hemiplegia or visual deficits in an AIDS patient	Progressive multifocal leukoencephalopathy (caused by JC virus)

What CNS infection commonly presents with fever, signs of ↑ ICP, focal neurologic signs, and a ring-enhancing lesion on CT?	Brain abscess

What are the organisms most commonly responsible for brain abscesses?	Anaerobes, gram-positive cocci, gram-negative rods
What is the recommended empiric antibiotic coverage for brain abscess?	Metronidazole and ceftriaxone (or another third generation cephalosporin)

Cognitive Disorders

Delirium or Dementia?

Waxing and waning level of consciousness	Delirium
Usually a rapid onset	Delirium
Characterized by **mem**ory loss	Dementia (Think De**MEM**tia)
Associated with disturbances in sleep-wake cycle	Delirium
Often irreversible	Dementia
Associated with changes in senso**rium** (hallucinations and illusions)	Delir**ium**
Name four major causes of delirium.	"HIDE" **H**ypoxia **I**nfection (often UTIs) and ICU psychosis **D**rugs (anticholinergics, opioids, steroids, barbiturates) **E**lectrolyte and **e**ndocrine causes
List four important steps in the evaluation of a patient with new-onset delirium.	1. Check vitals (including O_2 saturation) 2. Check med list 3. Check lab values 4. Check for occult infection
What is the treatment course for delirium?	Address underlying cause; neuroleptics for agitation
What cognitive disorder is characterized by progressive, global intellectual impairment?	Dementia
What is the most common etiology for dementia?	Dementia of Alzheimer Type (DAT) = 70–80% of cases

Name other common etiologies for dementia.

"DEMENTIASS"

Degenerative diseases (Parkinson's, Huntington's)

Endocrine (thyroid, pituitary, parathyroid)

Metabolic (electrolytes, glucose, hepatorenal dysfunction, ethanol)

Exogenous (CO poisoning, drugs, heavy metals)

Neoplastic

Traumatic

Infectious (encephalitis, meningitis, cerebral abscess, syphilis, prions, HIV, Lyme)

Affective disorders (depression may mimic dementia)

Stroke (multiinfarct dementia, ischemia, vasculitis); **Note:** Vascular causes account for 10% of dementias

Structural (normal pressure hydrocephalus [NPH]); **Note:** NPH is one of the few reversible causes of dementia

Name the type of dementia associated with the following features:

Associated with apolipoprotein E4 (ApoE4), amyloid precursor protein, presenilin, and α_2-macroglobulin genes

Alzheimer's

Risk for this type of dementia reduced with appropriate antihypertensive and antiplatelet medications

Vascular or multiinfarct

Cognitive impairment, extrapyramidal signs, and early visual hallucinations

Dementia with Lewy bodies

Insidious onset of difficulties with the activities of daily living and cognitive decline in the absence of other neurologic deficits

Alzheimer's

Stepwise dementia in a patient with focal neurologic deficits

Vascular or multiinfarct

Death occurs 5–10 years after the onset of cognitive decline	Alzheimer's
Dementia accompanied by changes in personality, speech disturbance, and extrapyramidal signs	Pick's
Triad of chorea, behavioral changes, and dementia	Huntington's
Most common cause of dementia; Donzepil may be helpful	Alzheimer's
Risk factors are identical to those of cerebrovascular disease	Vascular or multiinfarct
Difficulty with vertical gaze	Progressive supranuclear palsy
Rapidly progressive dementia associated with pyramidal, extrapyramidal and cerebellar motor decline, myoclonus, and increased startle response	Creutzfeldt-Jakob

Movement Disorders

Name the movement disorder associated with the following features:

Resting tremor, bradykinesia, rigidity, and postural instability → treat with dopamine (DA) replacement therapy	Parkinson's disease
Pediatric onset of sudden vocal or motor tics	Tourette's syndrome
Chorea, behavioral changes, and dementia	Huntington's disease
Postural tremor in the absence of other neurologic deficits	Essential tremor
Paroxysmal unilateral flailing limb movements	Hemiballism (2° to a lesion of the subthalamic nucleus)
Atrophy of the caudate and putamen	Huntington's disease
Tremor, ataxia, dysarthria, facial dystonia, parkinsonian signs, cognitive decline secondary to abnormal copper metabolism	Wilson's disease
Associated with schizophreniform changes	Huntington's disease

Amyotrophic Lateral Sclerosis, Multiple Sclerosis, and Other Demyelinating Diseases

What are the common symptoms of amyotrophic lateral sclerosis (ALS)?	Asymmetric, slowly progressive limb, bulbar weakness with fasciculations (i.e., difficulty swallowing)
What are the classic signs of ALS?	Upper motor neuron (UMN) signs (spasticity, hyperreflexia, clonus, upgoing toes, frontal reflexes) AND lower motor neuron (LMN) signs (flaccid paralysis, fasciculations)
What are the common EMG abnormalities in ALS?	Denervation potentials in at least three limbs
What is the common presentation of multiple sclerosis (MS)?	"Symptoms separated in time and space"; may include limb weakness, spasticity, optic nerve dysfunction, internuclear ophthalmoplegia, parasthesias, tremor, urinary retention, and vertigo
What are the classic radiologic abnormalities on magnetic resonance imaging (MRI) in a patient with MS?	Periventricular white matter lesions
What are the classic CSF abnormalities in a patient with MS?	Oligoclonal bands and mononuclear pleocytosis
What class of medications can be used during exacerbations?	Steroids
What class of medications can be used to prolong periods of remission?	Immunosuppressants (cyclophosphamide, azathioprine, methotrexate) and immunomodulators (β-interferon and copaxone)

Name the demyelinating disorder associated with the following clinical and pathologic features:

Most common demyelinating disorder	MS
Ascending paralysis, facial diplegia, and autonomic dysfunction	Guillain-Barré syndrome
Loss of myelin from globoid and peripheral neurons	Krabbe's disease
Charcot's triad (intention tremor, scanning speech, and nystagmus)	MS

Autosomal recessive (AR) disease → progressive paralysis, dementia, ataxia; fatal in early childhood	Metachromatic leukodystrophy
Spinal lesions typically occur in the white matter of the cervical cord	MS
Postviral autoimmune syndrome causing demyelination of peripheral nerves, especially motor fibers	Guillain-Barré syndrome
May present with intranuclear ophthalmoplegia (medial longitudinal fasciculus [MLF] syndrome) or sudden visual loss due to optic neuritis	MS
Albuminocytologic dissociation (↑ CSF protein with normal cell count)	Guillain-Barré syndrome
Rapidly fatal AR disease of childhood associated with globoid bodies in white matter due to deficiency of β-galactocerebrosidase	Krabbe's disease
Genetic disorder causing accumulation of very long chain fatty acids resulting in behavioral and a diverse array of changes neurologic deficits	Adrenoleukodystrophy

Vertigo

Name the vertiginous disorder associated with the following features:

Associated with popping sensation in the middle ear after sneezing, coughing, or straining	Endolymphatic fistula
Caused by head injury, may be associated with hearing loss	Labyrinthine concussion
Episodes of vertigo triggered by sudden changes in position; may be associated with recent trauma	Benign positional paroxysmal vertigo
Progressive hearing loss, episodic vertigo accompanied by nausea and vomiting and sense of fullness in the ear	Ménière's disease
Sudden onset of nausea, vomiting, and vertigo; self-limited disorder	Vestibular neuronitis

Vertical nystagmus, weakness, ataxia, CN palsies	Infarction of the vestibular system

Ophthalmology

Name the ophthalmologic disorder
with the following features:

Acute narrowing of anterior chamber angle associated with prolonged pupillary dilation	Angle closure glaucoma
Treatment includes ophthalmic artery thrombolysis	Central retinal artery occlusion
Sudden onset of blurred vision, eye pain; examination demonstrates a hard, red, painful eye with nonreactive pupil and increased intraocular pressure (IOP)	Angle closure glaucoma
Most common cause of permanent bilateral visual loss in the United States	Macular degeneration
Gradual increase in IOP with progressive eye pain, colored halos in visual field, and peripheral vision loss	Open angle glaucoma
Sudden, painless unilateral blindness; slowly reactive pupil and cherry red spot on fovea; associated with temporal arteritis	Central retinal artery occlusion
Must be treated emergently by lowering the IOP with acetazolamide; pilocarpine may be used once IOP is lowered	Angle closure glaucoma
More common in African Americans, age >40 y/o, and diabetics	Open angle glaucoma
Definitive therapy is laser iridotomy	Angle closure glaucoma
Loss of night and central vision; examination may show retinal pigment epithelium elevation or hemorrhagic changes	Macular degeneration
"Blood and thunder" appearance of fundus	Central retinal vein occlusion

MAKE THE DIAGNOSIS

55 y/o male presents with lower extremity weakness and muscle atrophy; physical examination (PE): ⊕ Babinski's sign, fasciculations, upper extremity hyperreflexia, and spasticity	Amyotrophic lateral sclerosis
65 y/o presents with a gradual decline in memory and inability to complete activities of daily living; Head CT: marked enlargement of ventricles and diffuse cortical atrophy	Alzheimer's disease
65 y/o female with h/o spinal metastases presents with pain radiating down the back of leg, saddle anesthesia, urinary retention; PE: absent ankle jerk reflexes; Lumbar CT: vertebral fracture with large bony fragment in lumbar spinal canal	Cauda equina syndrome
63 y/o male with h/o cartoid atherosclerosis presents with aphasia and right-sided weakness; PE: dense right hemiparesis, ⊕ Babinski's on right side	Left MCA cerebrovascular accident
20 y/o presents with nausea, vomiting, and headache 2 h after being hit in the temple with a baseball; patient lost consciousness initially but soon recovered; Head CT: lens-shaped, right-sided hyperdense mass adjacent to temporal bone	Epidural hematoma
40 y/o with h/o *Campylobacter* enteritis 1 week ago presents with ascending symmetric muscle weakness; PE: absent reflexes; W/U: CSF shows ↑ protein, normal cellular (albuminocytologic dissociation)	Guillain-Barré syndrome
37 y/o male presents with poor memory, depression, choreiform movements, and hypotonia; FH of a father who died at 45 after worsening tremors and dementia; Brain MRI: marked atrophy of the caudate nucleus	Huntington's disease

25 y/o with h/o bilateral temporal lobe contusions 1 week ago presents with a sudden increase in appetite, sexual desire, and hyperorality	Klüver-Bucy syndrome
30 y/o female with insidious onset of diplopia, scanning speech, parasthesias, numbness of right upper extremity, and urinary incontinence; W/U: CSF analysis is ⊕ for oligoclonal bands; MRI shows discrete areas of periventricular demyelination	MS
65 y/o female with h/o neurofibromatosis type 2 presents with headache, right-sided leg jerking, and worsening mental status; PE: papilledema and right-sided pronator drift; Head CT: dural-based, enhancing left-sided baseball-sized tumor	Meningioma
50 y/o with a h/o squamous cell carcinoma of the lung presents with N/V, headache, and diplopia; PE: papilledema, left oculomotor palsy, right pronator drift; Brain MRI: multiple round, ring-enhancing, hyperintense cortical, and cerebellar lesions	Metastases to brain
30 y/o female presents with unilateral throbbing headache, nausea, photophobia, and scotoma; similar symptoms occur monthly at the same time of her menstrual cycle	Migraine headache
62 y/o with urinary incontinence, loss of short-term memory, and dementia; PE: wide-based gate; head CT: massively dilated ventricular system	Normal pressure hydrocephalus
60 y/o presents with gradual onset of pill-rolling tremor; PE: masked facies, stooped posture, shuffling gait, cogwheel muscle rigidity	Parkinson's disease
31 y/o presents with loss of libido, galactorrhea, and irregular menses. PE: bitemporal hemianopia; W/U: negative β-hCG	Prolactinoma (Prolactin-secreting pituitary adenoma)

45 y/o presents with the gradual onset of sharp pain radiating from his buttocks down his leg that began 2 weeks ago while lifting a heavy box; PE: positive straight leg raise	Sciatica (2° to acute herniation of a lumbar disc)
50 y/o with h/o polycystic kidney disease presents with "worst headache of life," photophobia, nausea; PE: right eye deviates down and out; W/U: CSF is xanthrochromic	Subarachnoid hemorrhage (2° to ruptured berry aneurysm)
32 y/o male with h/o Arnold-Chiari malformation presents with bilateral upper extremity muscle weakness; PE: loss of pain and temperature sensation, ↓ DTR in upper extremities, and scoliosis; Spine MRI: central cavitation of the thoracic spinal cord	Syringomyelia
75 y/o alcoholic male on warfarin for h/o atrial fibrillation presents with declining mental status, headache, and papilledema; Head CT: crescenteric, hypodense 2 cm fluid collection along convexity of skull	Chronic subdural hematoma
30 y/o female with ⊕ FH for renal cell carcinoma presents with gait disturbance and blurred vision; PE: retinal hemangiomas, nystagmus, cerebellar ataxia, and dysdiadokinesia; Brain MRI: two cerebellar cystic lesions	von Hippel-Lindau disease
50 y/o with h/o alcoholism presents with psychosis, bilateral CN VI palsy, and ataxia; Brain MRI: mamillary body atrophy, periventricular hyperintensity on T2, and diffuse cortical atrophy	Wernicke's encephalopathy

## CHAPTER 4

Psychiatry

Describe the types of disorders that
fall under each of the following
DSM-IV classifications:

Axis I	Clinical psychiatric disorders
Axis II	Personality disorders and mental retardation
Axis III	Medical conditions
Axis IV	Social and environmental factors
Axis V	Global assessment of functioning (GAF)

Mood Disorders

What is the lifetime incidence of major
depressive disorder (MDD)?

Approximately 15%

Name the nine key features of MDD.

"SIG E CAPSS"

1. **S**leep changes
   (insomnia/hypersomnia)
2. **I**nability to experience pleasure,
   Interest ↓
3. **G**uilt or feelings of worthlessness
4. **E**nergy ↓ (fatigue)
5. **C**oncentration ↓, indecisiveness ↑
6. **A**ppetite disturbance with weight
   change (>5% body weight in
   1 month)
7. **P**sychomotor changes (agitation
   or retardation)
8. **S**uicidal ideations
9. **S**adness (depressed mood for
   most of the day)

What features are required to make the diagnosis for MDD?	**Two episodes** (involving five of the above nine—including #1 or #2) of impaired functioning for **2 week**, separated by **2 months**
What is in the differential diagnosis for a depressive disorder (d/o)?	MDD, bipolar d/o, dysthymia, secondary mood d/o, dementia, schizoaffective d/o, depressive d/o not otherwise specified (NOS), and bereavement (<2 months)
Name four sleep changes associated with MDD.	1. ↑ sleep latency 2. Early morning waking 3. ↓ stages 3 and 4 sleep 4. ↓ rapid eye movement (REM) latency and REM occurs earlier in the night
What type of depression, more common in children, is characterized by mood lability and rejection sensitivity?	Atypical depression
What class of drugs is commonly used first in the treatment of MDD?	Selective serotonin reuptake inhibitors (SSRIs)
Name two other classes of medication used for MDD.	Tricyclic antidepressants (TCAs) and monoamine oxidase inhibitors (MAOIs)
What is a safe, effective treatment for refractory MDD?	Electroconvulsive therapy (ECT)
What is the suicide rate in MDD?	Approximately 15–30%

Suicide

Name the risk factors for suicide.	**"SAD PERSONS"** **S**ex—male (women > attempts; men > actual suicides) **A**ge (bimodal: ↑ 15–24 and the elderly) **D**epression **P**revious attempts = #1 risk factor **E**thanol (and other substance abuse) **R**ational thought **S**ickness **O**rganized plan **N**o spouse **S**ocial support lacking

What is the approach to a patient who voices suicidal intentions?

Emergent inpatient hospitalization

Bipolar Disorder

What is the distinctively abnormal, irritable, elevated, expansive mood that lasts >1 week OR is severely impairing (e.g., requiring hospitalization)?

Manic episode

What are the seven key features of mania?

"DIG FAST" (at least three of following for diagnosis):

Distractibility

Insomnia

Grandiosity

Flight of ideas or racing thoughts

Psychomotor Agitation

Speech that is pressured or hyperverbal

Thoughtlessness (↑pleasurable activities → ↑consequences)

What is the differential diagnosis for bipolar d/o?

MDD, bipolars I and II, cyclothymia, schizoaffective d/o, borderline personality d/o, secondary mood d/o

What is the treatment for an acute manic episode?

First, manage agitation (benzos) and control mood (lithium, valproate, carbamazepine); then treat any psychoses

What is the treatment for bipolar depression?

Mood stabilizing drugs; ECT if refractory

Other Mood Disorders

Name the mood d/o associated with the following features:

Chronic d/o >2 years characterized by alternating hypomania and mild depression; absence of euthymia >2 months with no significant impairment

Cyclothymia

Less severe manic features present for several days that are NOT impairing; no psychotic features

Hypomania

History of major depressive episodes and at least one hypomanic episode	Bipolar II d/o
Manic episodes that may alternate with depressive episodes	Bipolar I d/o
Depressed mood for most of the day, for >50% of days, lasting >2 years with at least two signs of depression within last 2 months	Dysthymic d/o (**Note:** In kids diagnosis requires irritability and at least 1 year of ↓ mood)
Dysthymia plus MDD	Double depression
Name two types of secondary mood disorders.	1. Mood d/o due to medical condition (e.g., endocrinopathies, cancer, CNS infections) 2. Substance-induced mood d/o (i.e., steroids, reserpine, α-interferon ethanol, benzodiazepines). **Note:** Can be due to intoxication or withdrawal.

Psychotic Disorders

Give the appropriate term for each of the following psychotic symptoms:

False belief or wrong judgment held with conviction despite incontrovertible evidence to the contrary	Delusion
False perception of an actual external stimulus	Illusion
Thought d/o whereby ideas are not logically connected to those that occur before or after	Loose association
Misinterpreting others' actions or environmental cues as being directed toward one's self when, in fact, they are not	Idea of reference
Subjective perception of an object or event when no such external stimulus exists	Hallucination
What is the prevalence of schizophrenia?	0.9–1.2%
What is the risk of schizophrenia in primary relatives of a schizophrenic?	Siblings = 10%, parents of patient = 5.9%, kids of patient = 12.8%

What is the rate of suicide in schizophrenics?	10% at 10 years
What is the typical age of onset for schizophrenia?	Females = 25–35, males = 15–25
What is the differential for schizophrenia?	Schizoaffective d/o, schizophreniform d/o, brief psychotic d/o, delusional d/o, bipolar d/o, personality d/o, drug intoxication or withdrawal, and psychotic d/o due to a medical condition
Name the key features of schizophrenia.	Two or more psychotic symptoms for >1 month; impairment of social/occupational functioning; all >6 months
What are the guidelines for hospitalization for schizophrenia?	Hospitalize during psychotic episode if danger to self/others or unable to care for self
How is schizophrenia managed between psychotic episodes?	Treat antipsychotics and supportive psychotherapy; symptom monitoring
Give three examples of positive symptoms that are characteristic of schizophrenia.	Hallucinations, delusions, and disorganized thought processes (e.g., loose associations)
Positive symptoms respond best to what types of drugs?	Traditional antipsychotics (haloperidol)
Give four examples of negative symptoms that are characteristic of schizophrenia.	**The four As: A**ffect flattened, **A**logia, **A**nhedonia, **A**volition
Negative symptoms respond best to what types of drugs?	Atypical antipsychotics (clozapine, risperidone); Atypicals **for four A's**
Low-potency traditional antipsychotic agents are more likely to cause what types of side effects?	Anticholinergic, sedation, and hypotension
High-potency traditional antipsychotic agents are more likely to cause what types of side effects?	Neurologic (extrapyramidal symptoms [EPS], dystonia, tardive dyskinesia, and so on)
Name the DSM-IV subtype of schizophrenia associated with the following features:	
Delusions of persecution	Paranoid
Disinhibition; poor organization, personal appearance, and grooming	Disorganized (aka hebephrenic)

One previous schizophrenic episode with attenuated symptoms, but no active positive psychotic symptoms	Residual
Characteristics of more than one subtype	Undifferentiated
Bizarre posturing, mutism, stupor, *or* extreme excitability	Catatonic
Older age of onset, better functioning than other subtypes	Paranoid
Age of onset typically before 25 years	Disorganized

Name the psychotic d/o characterized by the following descriptions:

Psychotic symptoms lasting >1 day, but <1 month (often with obvious precipitating psychosocial stressor)	Brief psychotic d/o
Psychotic symptoms lasting 1–6 months	Schizophreniform d/o
Fixed, nonbizarre delusional system; without other thought disorders or impaired functioning	Delusional d/o
Symptoms of major mood d/o as well as of schizophrenia (with psychotic features occurring before mood disturbance); chronic social and occupational impairment	Schizoaffective d/o
Clouded consciousness, predominantly *visual* hallucinations, often occurring in inpatient setting	Psychotic d/o due to a general medical condition
Social withdrawal without psychosis	Schizoid personality d/o
Odd thought patterns (e.g., magical thinking) combined with peculiar behavior, without psychosis	Schizotypal personality d/o
Adopting the delusional system of a psychotic person	Shared psychotic d/o (Folie-à-deux)

Anxiety Disorders

What anxiety d/o is characterized by the recurrent, sudden-onset chest pain, tachypnea, nausea, trembling, and diaphoresis associated with fear (and lasts for 10 min)?	Panic d/o

What is the differential diagnosis for panic d/o?	Angina/myocardial infarction (MI), substance-induced anxiety, generalized anxiety d/o, posttraumatic stress disorder (PTSD), thyroid storm
What additional symptoms that follow these attacks are required to diagnose panic d/o?	Persistent concern about more attacks and worrying about the implications of the panic attacks
What phobia is often associated with panic d/o?	Agoraphobia
What medical conditions can be associated with panic d/o?	Mitral valve prolapse, hyperthyroidism, vitamin B_{12} deficiency, pheochromocytoma, arrhythmia
What anxiety d/o is characterized by marked, persistent fear of an object/situation which results in an unreasonable and excessive response, and thus the stimulus is avoided?	Specific phobia
What is the prevalence of specific phobias?	10–20% of the population (female >> males)
How does specific phobia differ from social phobia?	Unlike social phobia, specific phobia is a fear directed toward a specific object or situation
What is the treatment of choice for specific phobias?	Exposure therapy (e.g., desensitization, flooding)
What anxiety d/o can occur after a person is subjected to a traumatic event?	PTSD
Name the five major criteria for diagnosing PTSD.	1. Exposure to a traumatic event causing intense fear or horror 2. Reexperiencing the event (in dreams, flashbacks, and so on) 3. Avoiding stimuli related to the trauma and overall "numbing" of responsiveness 4. Symptoms of hyperarousal/hypervigilance 5. Clinically significant impairment
What two traumatic events are *most likely* to cause PTSD in males and females?	**Males:** Rape > combat **Females:** Childhood abuse > rape
What often complicates the treatment of PTSD?	Substance abuse

What is the treatment approach for PTSD? | First, address any underlying substance abuse; SSRIs (fluoxetine) and MAOIs (phenelzine); β-blockers for autonomic symptoms; behavioral therapy and support groups

What anxiety d/o is characterized by symptoms of PTSD that occur within 4 weeks of the stressor and last <4 weeks? | Acute stress d/o

What anxiety d/o is characterized by excessive worrying for >50% of the days over the past 6 months that causes significant impairment? | Generalized anxiety d/o; prevalence = 4–9% (females >> males)

What is the treatment of choice for generalized anxiety d/o? | Intermediate-acting benzodiazepines (less addiction, last reasonably long) or buspirone (preferable in those with addiction potential)

What anxiety d/o is characterized by maladaptive behavioral symptoms related to an identifiable stressor, which occurs *within 3 months* of a traumatic incident and results in functional impairment? | Adjustment d/o

What term is used to describe recurrent, intrusive, senseless thoughts, images, and impulses? | Obsessions

What term is used to describe repetitive behaviors driven by the conscious will to respond to an obsession and thereby decrease the anxiety caused by it? | Compulsions

Name three common obsessions. | Contamination, symmetry, fear of being harmed (or harming others)

Name three common compulsions. | Cleaning, Checking, Counting (The three Cs of Compulsion)

Name two ways in which obsessive-compulsive disorder (OCD) differs from obsessive-compulsive personality type. | 1. The d/o causes significant distress and impaired functioning.
2. Patients are aware that their behaviors are unreasonable, but are not able to control them.

What is the treatment of choice for OCD? | SSRIs (fluvoxamine) or TCAs (clomipramine), and cognitive-behavioral therapy

Somatoform Disorders

What somatoform d/o is characterized by multiple, unrelated physical complaints leading to excessive medical attention seeking and severely impaired functioning?

Somatization disorder
(females:males = 5:1)

What combination of complaints fulfills the diagnostic criteria for somatization d/o?

Complaints of four pain, two GI, one sexual/GU, and one pseudoneurologic symptoms; **Note:** Cannot be intentional or fake

Name the somatoform d/o characterized by the following descriptions:

Prolonged preoccupation with concerns of having a serious illness (despite negative medical workups) and exaggerated attention to bodily or mental sensations

Hypochondriasis

Conscious simulation of physical or psychologic illness solely to receive attention from medical personnel

Factitious d/o (Munchausen's syndrome); **Note:** Technically NOT a somatoform d/o because it is intentional

Intentionally simulating illness for personal gain (usually financial)

Malingering; **Note:** Also NOT a somatoform d/o; suspect in cases involving litigation

Preoccupation with an imagined physical defect, causing significantly impaired social and occupational functioning

Body dysmorphic disorder (BDD)

Sudden onset of motor/sensory neurologic d/o following a traumatic emotional event

Conversion d/o

What eating d/o is characterized by refusal to maintain normal body weight and extreme fear of becoming obese, resulting in life-threatening weight loss?

Anorexia nervosa; prevalence = 1% in adolescent females (90% of cases are female)

Name four important features in the patient history that suggest anorexia nervosa.

Distorted body image (perceive self as being fat), >15% below ideal body weight, amenorrhea, excessive exercise

What tests should be included in the workup of anorexia nervosa?	Accurate height/weight measurements, ECG, electrolytes, CBC, total protein, βhCG, thyroid tests, and psychiatric evaluation
What is the appropriate management of anorexia nervosa?	1. Correct nutritional/electrolyte status 2. Psychotherapy 3. Monitor weight, food/calorie intake, and urine output
What is the mortality rate in anorexia nervosa?	Six to twenty percent
What eating d/o is characterized by episodes of binge eating associated with emotional distress and accompanied by compensatory behaviors aimed at preventing weight gain?	Bulimia nervosa
Name five compensatory behaviors that patients employ to prevent weight gain from bingeing.	Self-induced vomiting, diuretic abuse, laxative abuse, use of appetite suppressants, and/or medications intended to speed up the metabolism (e.g., thyroid hormone)
Name four important features in the patient history that suggest bulimia nervosa.	Distorted body image, relatively normal body weight, avoid eating around others, morbid preoccupation with food/eating that leads to binge eating episodes
Name three physical examination findings that may suggest bulimia nervosa.	Bilateral parotid enlargement, periodontal disease or extensive dental erosions, and Russel's sign
What is Russel's sign?	Scarring and abrasions on the knuckles from repeated self-induced vomiting
What is the treatment course for bulimia nervosa?	Cognitive-behavioral therapy and SSRIs
What antidepressant is contraindicated in bulimia?	Bupropion (Wellbutrin)—↑ risk of seizures

Substance Abuse

What is the lifetime prevalence of substance abuse/dependence?	~13%

Name four classic signs of substance abuse.

1. Recurrent use causing failure of work, school, or home obligations
2. Recurrent substance-related legal issues
3. Recurrent use in physically hazardous situations
4. Continued use in spite of consequences of use

How is "dependence" defined?

Withdrawal occurs if substance is stopped and patient has tolerance to substance

Not counting tobacco and caffeine, what is the most commonly abused substance in the United States?

Alcohol

What is a short, useful screening tool for alcoholism?

"CAGE" questions

Have you felt the need to Cut down?

Have you ever felt Annoyed by criticism of your drinking?

Have you ever felt Guilty about drinking?

Have you ever had an Eye opener?

What is the major complication of alcohol withdrawal and when is it most likely to occur?

Delirium tremens (DTs); peak occurrence is 2–7 days. **Note:** DTs are a medical emergency

What is the mortality rate of DTs?

15–20%

What is the medical management of alcohol withdrawal?

Benzodiazepine taper for symptoms; haloperidol for hallucinations; thiamine, folate, and multivitamin replacement; correct electrolyte abnormalities; eventual group therapy or 12-step program

Name three GI complications of alcoholism.

GI bleeding (from ulcers, gastritis, esophageal varices, or Mallory-Weiss tears), pancreatitis, and liver disease

What syndrome of anterograde amnesia, confabulations, ataxia, and nystagmus results from chronic alcoholism?

Wernicke-Korsakoff syndrome

What am I high on?

CNS and respiratory depression, euphoria, pinpoint pupils, nausea, and ↓ GI motility

Opioids (goosebumps → *cold turkey*); inspect for track marks along veins

Psychomotor agitation, dilated pupils, euphoria, ↑ heart rate (HR) and BP, prolonged wakefulness and attention, delusions, ↑ pain threshold	Amphetamines
All of the above, plus tactile hallucinations, angina, and sudden cardiac death	Cocaine
Intense violence, psychosis, and delirium; psychomotor agitation, nystagmus, ataxia; rhabdomyolysis and hyperthermia	Phencyclidine hydrochloride (PCP)
Delusions, visual hallucinations, postuse flashbacks	Lysergic acid diethylamide (LSD)
Disinhibition, emotional lability, slurred speech, ataxia, blackouts, coma	Alcohol

What am I coming down from and how is it treated?

Anxiety and "flu-like symptoms" (insomnia, piloerection, fever, rhinorrhea, yawning, ↑ GI motility)	Opioids → naltrexone/naloxone for overdose; methadone for detoxification
Recurrence of sudden-onset, homicidal violence, and psychosis	PCP → antipsychotics and benzodiazepines
Hypersomnolence, fatigue, depression, malaise, severe craving for drug (peaks 2–4 days after last dose)	Cocaine → haloperidol, benzodiazepines, antiemetics, antiinflammatory (for myalgias); bromocriptine for withdrawal
Postuse "crash" (lethargy, headache, hunger, depression, dysphoric mood, altered sleep)	Amphetamines → similar to cocaine
Tremor, ↑ HR and BP, malaise, nausea, seizures, agitation, delirium	Alcohol → (see above)

Childhood Disorders

Name the d/o of childhood described by each of the following statements:

Repetitive behaviors (in patient <18 y/o) that violate social norms; may exhibit physical aggression, cruelty to animals, vandalism and robbery, along with truancy, cheating, and lying	Conduct d/o (Remember: predominantly *actions*)

Recurrent pattern of negativistic, hostile, and disobedient behavior toward authority figures; loss of temper and defiance (but not theft lying)	Oppositional defiant d/o or (Remember: predominantly *words*)
Developmentally inappropriate degrees of inattention, impulsiveness, and hyperactivity at home, in school, and in social situations; present *before age 7*	Attention-deficit hyperactivity disorder (ADHD)
Pervasive developmental disorder (PDD) with stereotyped movements and nonprogressive impairments in social interactions, communication, and behavior	Autism
Progressive syndrome of autism, dementia, ataxia, and purposeless hand movements; associated with hyperammonemia; principally in girls	Rett syndrome
PDD with severe impairment in social skills and repetitive behaviors, leading to impaired social and occupational functioning but without significant delays in language development	Asperger d/o

Name three findings that are suggestive of each type of abuse listed below:

Physical child abuse	Healed fractures at different stages, cigarette burns, retinal hemorrhage/ detachment (32% of kids <5 y/o are physically abused)
Sexual child abuse	Genital/anal trauma, STDs, UTIs (25% of kids <8 y/o are sexually abused)
Elder abuse	Evidence of depleted finances, poor hygiene, spiral fractures

Personality Disorders

Name four qualities that distinguish a personality d/o from a personality *trait*.	1. Maladaptive 2. Enduring (lifelong) 3. Inflexible 4. Impairs social/occupational functioning

List the three cluster A personality disorders.

"Weird"

1. Paranoid
2. Schizoid
3. Schizotypal

List the four cluster B personality disorders.

"Wild"

1. Histrionic
2. Borderline
3. Antisocial
4. Narcissistic

List the three cluster C personality disorders.

"Worried"

1. Avoidant
2. Obsessive-compulsive
3. Dependent

Name the personality d/o characterized by each of the following statements:

Social inhibition, sensitive to rejection, inferiority complex

Avoidant (C)

Peculiar appearance, interpersonal awkwardness, "magical" or odd thought patterns, no psychosis

Schizotypal (A)

Impulsive, unstable mood, chaotic relationships, sense of feeling empty and alone, self-mutilation, females >> males

Borderline (B)

Sense of entitlement, grandiosity, lack empathy for others, insists on special treatment when ill

Narcissistic (B)

Suspicious and distrustful, uses projection as primary defense mechanism

Paranoid (A)

Lacks self-confidence, submissive, and clingy

Dependent (C)

Unable to maintain intimate relationships, extroverted, melodramatic, sexually provocative

Histrionic (B)

Disregards and violates rights of others, criminality, males > females; <18 y/o = conduct d/o

Antisocial (B)

Lifelong pattern of voluntary social withdrawal, no psychosis, shows minimal emotions

Schizoid (A)

PSYCHOPHARMACOLOGY

Antidepressants

For each of the following drugs, provide:
(1) the mechanism of action (MOA),
(2) indication(s) (IND), and (3) significant
side effects and unique toxicity (TOX)
(if any):

TCAs (imipramine, clomipramine, amitriptyline, desipramine, nortriptyline, doxepin, amoxapine)

MOA: Prevents reuptake of norepinephrine (NE) and 5-hydroxytryptamine (5-HT)

IND: Depression, enuresis (imipramine), depression in elderly (nortriptyline), OCD (clomipramine), depression with psychotic features (amoxapine), fibromyalgia

TOX: Sedation (desipramine is least sedating), anticholinergic effects, lethal in overdose → respiratory depression, hyperpyrexia, and **TriCs**: **C**ardiac arrhythmia, **C**onvulsions, **C**oma

SSRIs (fluoxetine, paroxetine, sertraline, citalopram, fluvoxamine, escitalopram)

MOA: Selectively blocks reuptake of 5-HT (usually requires 2–3 weeks to take effect)

IND: Depression, premenstrual syndrome (flouxetine), OCD (fluvoxamine)

TOX: Agitation, insomnia, sexual dysfunction, "Serotonin syndrome" with MAOIs (muscle rigidity, hyperthermia, cardiovascular collapse)

Bupropion

MOA: Heterocyclic agent, mechanism not well known

IND: Depression, smoking cessation

TOX: Agitation, seizures, insomnia (↓ sexual side effects)

Trazodone

MOA: Mainly inhibits serotonin reuptake

IND: Depression

TOX: Postural hypotension, sedation, priapism

Venlafaxine	**MOA:** Inhibits 5-HT and NE reuptake
	IND: Depression, generalized anxiety d/o
	TOX: Stimulant effects, minimal effects on P450
Mirtazapine	**MOA:** $5\text{-}HT_2$ receptor antagonist and α_2-antagonist $\rightarrow \uparrow$ NE and 5-HT release
	IND: Depression
	TOX: Sedation, $\uparrow$ appetite, $\uparrow$ cholesterol
MAOIs **(TIP:** Tranylcypromine, Isocarboxazid, Phenelzine)	**MOA:** Nonselective MAOIs
	IND: Atypical depressions, anxiety disorders, pain disorders, eating disorders
	TOX: Hypertensive crisis with tyramine or meperidine ingestion, Serotonin syndrome with SSRIs
Lithium	**MOA:** Prevents generation of (IP_3) and (DAG) 2° messenger systems
	IND: Bipolar d/o (prevents and treats acute mania)
	TOX: Hypothyroidism, nephrogenic diabetes insipidus (DI), teratogenesis (Ebstein anomaly)

Antipsychotics

What is the name for stereotyped oral-facial movements that occur as a result of long-term antipsychotic use?	Tardive dyskinesia
Describe the chronology of extrapyramidal side effects from neuroleptic medications.	"**Rule of fours:**" 4 h—acute dystonia, 4 days— akinesia, 4 weeks—akathesia, 4 months— tardive dyskinesia (usually irreversible)
What is the characteristic triad of neuroleptic malignant syndrome (NMS)?	Muscle rigidity, autonomic instability, and hyperpyrexia
What is the treatment for NMS?	Dantrolene and dopamine agonists

For each of the following drugs, provide: (1) the mechanism of action (MOA), (2) indication(s) (IND), and (3) significant side effects and unique toxicity (TOX) (if any):

Traditional high-potency antipsychotics (haloperidol, perphenazine, trifluoperazine)

MOA: D_2 dopamine receptors antagonists (also block α_2, muscarinic, and histaminic receptors)

IND: Schizophrenia, psychosis (especially positive symptoms)

TOX: ↑ neurologic (e.g., extrapyramidal) side effects (SEs), NMS, tardive dyskinesia

Traditional low-potency antipsychotics (chlorpromazine, thioridazine)

MOA: D_2 dopamine receptor antagonists (also block α_2, muscarinic, and histaminic receptors)

IND: Schizophrenia, psychosis

TOX: ↓ neurologic SEs, ↑ anticholinergic and endocrine SEs; cardiac conduction defects and retinal pigmentation (thioridazine), corneal and lenticular deposits (chlorpromazine)

Atypical antipsychotics (clozapine, risperidone, olanzapine, quetiapine)

MOA: $5\text{-}HT_2$ antagonists; D_4 and $D_1 > D_2$ receptor antagonists

IND: Schizophrenia, psychosis (especially *negative* symptoms); OCD/anxiety d/o (olanzapine)

TOX: ↓ anticholinergic and EPS, ↑ hematologic SEs; agranulocytosis (clozapine → weekly WBC monitoring)

Name the drug of choice in each of the following clinical settings:

Depression with insomnia; chronic pain

Amitriptyline (Elavil)

OCD

Clomipramine (Anafranil) or fluvoxamine (Luvox)

Depression with anorexia nervosa or bulimia

Desipramine (Norpramin)— stimulates appetite

Depression with psychotic features

Amoxapine (Asendin)

Refractory psychosis with predominantly negative symptoms

Clozapine (Clozaril)

Panic d/o with agoraphobia	Imipramine (Tofranil)
ADHD in children	Methylphenidate (Ritalin, Concerta, Methylin)
Adult ADHD	Bupropion (Wellbutrin, Zyban)
Premenstrual dysmorphic d/o	Fluoxetine (Paxil)
Trichotillomania	Clomipramine (Anafranil)
Intractable hiccups, with nausea and vomiting	Chlorpromazine (Thorazine)
MDD	Fluoxetine (Paxil)
Anxiety in the elderly	Buspirone (BuSpar)—less sedating
Tourette d/o	Pimozide (Orap)
Alcohol withdrawal symptoms	Chlordiazepozide (Librium)
Smoking cessation	Bupropion (Wellbutrin, Zyban)
Generalized anxiety d/o	Venlafexine (Effexor) or buspirone (BuSpar)
Enuresis	Imipramine (Tofranil)
Used to decrease alcohol dependence	Disulfiram (Antabuse) and naltrexone (ReVia)
Panic attacks	Clonazepam (Klonopin)
Overdose with benzodiazepines	Flumazenil (Romazicon)
Hypertensive crisis from tyramine and MAOIs	Phentolamine
Atypical depression	MAOIs (e.g., Phenelzine)

List the *unique* toxicities of the following psychiatric drugs:

TCAs	"Three Cs:" Convulsions, Cardiac Arrhythmias, Coma
Trazodone (Desyrel)	Priapism
Clozapine (Clozaril)	Agranulocytosis—monitor CBCs weekly; seizures
MAOIs	Hyperadrenergic/hypertensive crisis (with tyramine)
Lithium (Eskalith)	Nephrogenic DI, hypothyroidism, teratogenesis

Thioridazine (Mellaril)	Cardiac conduction abnormalities, irreversible retinal pigmentation
Chlorpromazine (Thorazine)	Corneal and lenticular deposits, NMS
Fluphenazine (Prolixin)	Hepatotoxicity, NMS
Carbamazepine (Tegretol)	Aplastic anemia, hepatoxicity
Valproate (Depakene)	Hepatotoxicity (rare, but lethal), syndrome of inappropriate antidiuretic hormone secretion (SIADH), Stevens-Johnson syndrome, teratogenesis
Lamotrigine (Lamictal)	Stevens-Johnson syndrome, toxic epidermal necrolysis
Haloperidol (Haldol)	Arrhythmias (including torsades), NMS
Name the short-acting benzodiazepines.	"TOM is Short" Triazolam (Halcion) Oxazepam (Serax) Midazolam (Versed)
Name the intermediate-acting benzodiazepines.	"TALC" Temazepam (Restoril) Alprazolam (Xanax) Lorazepam (Ativan) Clonazepam (Klonopin)
Name the long-acting benzodiazepines.	"CD" Chlordiazepoxide (Librium) Diazepam (Valium)
Name the benzodiazepines acceptable for use in patients with hepatic dysfunction (Note: These agents are not metabolized by liver and are excreted by kidneys.)	"LOT" Lorazepam (Ativan) Oxazepam (Serax) Temazepam (Restoril) **Note:** Chlordiazepoxide (Librium) often used for DTs if no evidence of hepatic dysfunction

MAKE THE DIAGNOSIS

20 y/o female presents with excessive anxiety about a variety of events for more than half of the days for the last 7 months	Generalized anxiety d/o
68 y/o veteran presents with complaints of vivid flashbacks, hypervigilance, and difficulty falling asleep for the past several years; PE: patient appears very anxious	Posttraumatic stress d/o
28 y/o male who systematically checks each lock in his house multiple times before leaving, often causing him to be over an hour late for meetings	Obsessive-compulsive d/o (OCD)
29 y/o male presents with a 9-month h/o insatiable urges to rub himself against strangers, which he has regrettably acted upon several times	Frotteurism (sexual paraphilia)
22 y/o female college student who is 20% below her ideal body weight complains of not having any menstrual cycles and "feeling fat"	Anorexia nervosa
26 y/o female medical student for the past 9 months is convinced she has systemic lupus erythematosus (SLE) and despite numerous negative workups, she fears she will have to drop out of school	Hypochondriasis
17 y/o female presents with complaints of "feeling fat" and h/o eating dinner alone in her bedroom; PE: normal height and weight, dental erosions, and ⊕ Russel's sign	Bulimia
24 y/o with h/o depression presents with inability to sleep, and auditory hallucinations; PE: easy distractibility and pressured speech; W/U: normal TSH and negative toxicology screen	Bipolar d/o (manic episode)
21 y/o female with no h/o trauma presents to the ER because she cannot feel or move her legs; W/U: completely within normal limits (WNL); detailed history reveals that her boyfriend of 8 years left her this morning	Conversion d/o

43 y/o alcoholic with h/o confabulation and amnesia presents to ER after falling down; PE: nystagmus and ataxic gait; W/U: macrocytic anemia	Wernicke-Korsakoff syndrome
6 y/o presents with 8 month h/o hyperactivity, inattentiveness, and impulsivity both at school and at home; PE and W/U are essentially WNL	ADHD
33 y/o female presents to your office distressed after turning down a lucrative job offer because of the requirement to speak in front of people	Social phobia
9 y/o boy with 2-year h/o involuntary tics is brought to your office because he has recently been shouting obscenities	Tourette's syndrome
33 y/o female nurse presents with recent occurrences of hypoglycemia; PE: reveals multiple crossed scars on abdomen; W/U: insulin/C-peptide ratio >1.0	Factitious d/o (Munchausen's syndrome)
16 y/o with h/o sudden-onset daytime sleep attacks with loss of muscle tone and audiovisual hallucinations while waking and falling asleep	Narcolepsy
19 y/o with 8 month h/o deteriorating grades and social withdrawal presents with auditory hallucinations; PE: odd thinking patterns, tangential thoughts, and flattened affect; W/U: negative toxicology screen	Schizophrenia
48 y/o female presents with recent h/o early morning waking, ↓ appetite, feelings of guilt, and loss of interest in her usual hobbies over the past 3 months; PE and labs are WNL	Major depressive d/o
3 y/o male with h/o of poor cuddling presents with severely delayed language and social development; PE: below normal intelligence with unusual calculating abilities, and repetitive behaviors	Autism

## CHAPTER 5

Obstetrics and Gynecology

OBSTETRICS

Complete the following formulas:

Gestational age (GA)/estimated date of confinement (EDC) =	Age of fetus from last menstrual period
# of live births/1000 people =	Birthrate
# of live births/1000 females 15–44 years old =	Fertility rate
# of neonatal deaths/1000 live births =	Neonatal mortality rate
# of stillbirths + neonatal deaths/1000 total births =	Perinatal mortality rate
# of infant deaths/1000 live births up to first year of life =	Infant mortality rate

Diagnosis of Pregnancy

What are typical signs and symptoms of early pregnancy?	Amenorrhea, nausea, vomiting (N/V), breast tenderness, **Chadwick's sign** (bluish discoloration and congested appearance of vagina), and **Hegar's sign** (softening of lower segment of uterus)
At what GA can fetal heart tones (FHT) be detected by Doppler?	10 weeks
At what GA can the ultrasound (U/S) detect a gestational sac and cardiac activity?	5 weeks and after 6 weeks, respectively

Name the three signs of fetal viability during pregnancy.	1. Fetal heart activity 2. Fetal movement detection by examiner 3. Embryo/fetus ultrasonic recognition
How early can human chorionic gonadotropin (βhCG) be detected in urine or serum?	As early as 8–9 days after ovulation
What is the doubling time of βhCG in early pregnancy?	2 days
When does βhCG peak in pregnancy?	Eight to 10 weeks GA
Name three clinical scenarios in which quantification of βhCG is helpful.	1. Diagnosing ectopic pregnancy 2. Monitoring neoplastic trophoblastic disease 3. Screening fetal aneuploidy

Dating

What is Nägele's rule?	EDC = LMP + 7 days − 3 months + 1 year (based on regular 28-day cycle)
What is the most common cause of size-for-dates discrepancy?	Inaccurate dating

Physiologic Changes in Pregnancy

What are the physiologic changes of pregnancy in the following systems?	
Cardiovascular	↑ heart rate (HR) and SV → ↑ CO; systolic ejection murmur (SEM) is normal finding; diastolic murmur is NEVER a normal finding; ↓ BP (especially diastolic)—lowest at 24 weeks
Respiratory	↑ tidal volume and minute ventilation, ↓ total lung capacity (elevation of diaphragm), ↑ total body O_2 consumption, and hyperventilation (optimizes CO_2 and O_2 transfer between mother and fetus)
Gastrointestinal	N/V, reflux esophagitis, hemorrhoids, and cholestasis

Renal	↑ Glomerular filtration rate (GFR) 50%, ↓ BUN and Cr, urinary stasis, and asymptomatic bacteriuria in ~5%
Hematologic	↓ Hematocrit (Hct): ↑ plasma volume by 40% (due to ↑ plasma > RBC); hypercoagulable state: ↑ clotting factors (↓ protein S), ↑ venous stasis, and endothelial damage
Dermatologic	↑ estrogen → spider angiomata and palmar erythema; ↑ melanocyte stimulating hormone → hyperpigmentation of nipples, abdominal midline (linea nigra), and face (chloasma/melasma)
Endocrine	↑ hCG, human placental lactogen (hPL—insulin antagonist with diabetogenic effect), progesterone, estrogen, thyroid binding globulin, T3 and T4 (euthyroid state), and prolactin

General Prenatal Care

What labs should be obtained at the first prenatal visit?	CBC, Rh factor, antibody screen, Pap smear, gonorrhea, and Chlamydia cultures, urinalysis (UA) and culture, rubella, syphilis, hepatitis B, HIV, TB
Why is folate an essential part of prenatal vitamins?	Proven to ↓ risk of neural tube defects (NTD)

Teratogens

At what GA are structural abnormalities most likely to occur as a result of teratogens?	3–8 weeks since conception (organogenesis phase)
Name the teratogenic effects of the following substances:	
Angiotensin converting enzyme inhibitors (ACEi)	Renal dysgenesis → oligohydramnios, pulmonary hypoplasia and limb contractures

Tetracycline	Discolored teeth and enamel hypoplasia
Aminogylcosides	Acoustic nerve damage $\rightarrow$ deafness
Oral hypoglycemics	Neonatal hypoglycemia
Dilantin	Fetal hydantoin syndrome: craniofacial and limb defects, mental deficiencies
Valproic acid	Spina bifida
Isotretinoin	Craniofacial (small ears), central nervous system (CNS), cardiac, and thymus defects
Indomethacin	Constriction of ductus arteriosus
Diethylstilbesterol (DES)	Clear cell vaginal cancer and cervical/uterine malformations in female offspring
Thalidomide	Limb reduction defects
Alcohol	Fetal alcohol syndrome: craniofacial defects (absent philtrum, flattened nasal bridge, microphthalmia), growth restriction, brain, cardiac, and spinal defects
Tobacco	Growth restriction
Radiation	Growth restriction, CNS defects, leukemia

ANTEPARTUM

Medical Conditions in Pregnancy

Gestational Diabetes Mellitus (GDM)

What is the prevalence of GDM?	~7% of pregnancies; **Note:** Most common medical complication of pregnancy
What are five risk factors for GDM?	1. >25 y/o 2. Obesity 3. ⊕ family history (FH) of diabetes mellitus (DM) 4. Previous infant >4000 g 5. Previous (h/o) polyhydramnios

How is GDM diagnosed?

Screened with glucose challenge test (50 g glucose); diagnosed with glucose tolerance test (100 g)

What are four components of GDM management?

1. American Dietetic Association (ADA) diet; insulin if necessary
2. Avoid oral hypoglycemics
3. U/S for fetal growth assessment
4. Nonstress test (NST) starting at 30–32 weeks

What is the White Classification for GDM?

A1: diet controlled, A2: insulin requiring

What percentage of women with GDM will develop overt DM after their pregnancy?

>50%

Preexisting Diabetes Mellitus

How is preexisting DM managed?

Insulin, monitor Hgb_{A1c}, U/S, and maternal serum alpha-fetoprotein (MSAFP) check at 16–20 weeks, fetal echocardiogram at 20 weeks, twice weekly NST starting at 30–32 weeks

When should elective cesarean section (c/s) be considered in a patient with DM?

Fetal weight >4500 g (may consider elective delivery at 36–38 weeks with evidence of fetal lung maturity)

What are the maternal complications of DM?

Preeclampsia/eclampsia (twofold ↑ risk), hyperglycemia, retinopathy, diabetic ketoacidosis (DKA)

What are the fetal complications of DM?

Macrosomia (>4500 g), cardiac defects, caudal regression (malformations associated with poor glucose control), polyhydramnios, hypoglycemia secondary ($2°$) to hyperinsulinemia, IUFD

What are the obstetrical complications of DM?

Preterm labor (PTL) and shoulder dystocia

Hypertension in Pregnancy

Name the hypertensive disorder (d/o) of pregnancy described below:

BP ≥140/90 before pregnancy or diagnosed before 20 weeks GA

Chronic hypertension (HTN)

BP 140/90–160/110, proteinuria 300–5000 mg/24 h, or 1–2+ on dipstick

Preeclampsia (mild)

BP >160/110, proteinuria >5000 mg/24 h, or 3–4+ on dipstick	Preeclampsia (severe)
Preeclampsia with seizures	Eclampsia
Define the **HELLP** syndrome.	Hemolytic anemia, Elevated (LFTs), Low Platelets
What are other signs and symptoms of severe preeclampsia/eclampsia?	Headache (HA), blurred vision, epigastric pain, hyperreflexia, and clonus
What are the risk factors for preeclampsia?	Multifetal gestation, nulliparity, ⊕ FH, maternal age <20 or >35 y/o, chronic HTN, African American
What is the management of mild preeclampsia with immature fetus?	Bed rest and monitoring of BP, weight, and 24° urine protein levels
What is the management of severe preeclampsia and eclampsia?	Magnesium sulfate ($MgSO_4$) until 12–24 h postpartum (PP), ↓ BP, and delivery; if fetal or maternal deterioration at any gestational age → **induce labor** (delivery is the definitive treatment)
What percentage of maternal mortalities are due to pulmonary embolism?	10% (#1 cause of maternal death)
What is the treatment for DVT or pulmonary embolism in pregnancy?	Heparin or low molecular weight heparin (**never warfarin!**)
What is the drug of choice for hyperthyroidism in pregnancy?	Propylthiouracil (PTU) in Pregnancy
Why should asymptomatic bacteriuria be treated in pregnant women?	25% will develop acute, symptomatic infection if untreated
What is the most common cause of septic shock in pregnancy?	Acute pyelonephritis
What is the management of acute pyelonephritis?	*Hospitalization*, urine and blood culture, IV hydration, IV ABX, urine culture 1–2 weeks after completion of treatment/therapy (test of cure)
What is the minimum medical treatment for HIV ⊕ pregnant women?	Azidothymidine (AZT) after 14 weeks GA through labor for mom; AZT for newborn
What is the rate of vertical transmission of HIV on AZT prophylaxis?	~8% (↓ from 25% without prophylaxis)

What mode of delivery is recommended if the HIV viral load >1000 at 36 weeks GA?	Scheduled c/s
What mode of delivery is recommended in a pregnant woman with active herpes lesions during the intrapartum period?	C/s
When is universal GBS screening performed?	36 weeks GA
What anatomy must be swabbed for a complete GBS culture?	Lower vagina and rectum (through sphincter)
What is the drug of choice for GBS positive patients during the intrapartum period?	Penicillin
What is chorioamnionitis and how is it treated?	Infection of the amniotic fluid (most common cause of neonatal sepsis); broad-spectrum ABX and delivery

Obstetrical Complications

What is the differential diagnosis for bleeding in the first trimester?	Ectopic pregnancy, spontaneous abortion (SAB), postcoital bleeding, vaginal/cervical lesion, molar pregnancy, nonobstetric cause

Ectopic Pregnancy

What is the definition of an ectopic pregnancy?	Pregnancy outside uterine cavity (95% occur in the fallopian tubes)
What are five risk factors for ectopic pregnancy?	1. h/o pelvic inflammatory disease (PID) or prior ectopic 2. Pelvic surgery 3. DES exposure in utero 4. Intrauterine device (IUD) usage 5. Endometriosis
What is the clinical triad of ectopic pregnancy?	1. Amenorrhea 2. Abdominal pain 3. Irregular vaginal bleeding
Name three *signs* of a ruptured ectopic pregnancy.	Hypotension, tachycardia, and rebound tenderness
What is the differential diagnosis for suspected ectopic pregnancy?	Surgical abdomen, abortion, ovarian torsion, and ruptured ovarian cyst

What are four methods used to diagnose ectopic pregnancy?	1. Positive pregnancy test with empty uterus by U/S 2. Prolonged hCG doubling 3. Progesterone <25 ng/mL 4. Surgical abdomen
What medical treatment is indicated in stable, unruptured ectopic pregnancy <3.5 cm and <6 weeks GA?	Methotrexate
What is the treatment for most other ectopic pregnancies?	Laparoscopic surgery

Abortion

Define spontaneous abortion (SAB) or miscarriage.	Loss of pregnancy before 20 weeks GA or delivery of fetus <500 g
Name the type of abortion described below (all <20 weeks GA) and appropriate treatment:	
Intrauterine bleeding *without* dilation of cervix and no expulsion of products of conception (POC)	Threatened **Tx:** After documenting a live fetus, bed rest and pelvic rest.
Intrauterine bleeding *with* dilation of cervix and no expulsion of POC	Inevitable **Tx:** Surgical evacuation of uterine contents.
Partial expulsion of POC	Incomplete **Tx:** Hospitalization, possible hemodynamic resuscitation, and curettage
Complete expulsion of POC	Complete **Tx:** None
Death of embryo/fetus with retention of POC	Missed **Tx:** Surgical evacuation of uterine contents if there is no spontaneous resolution
≥2 consecutive or three total SAB	Recurrent **Tx:** Based on type of abortion
What is the most common cause of a first trimester fetal death?	Chromosomal abnormality
What are signs/symptoms of SAB?	Vaginal bleeding, cramping, abdominal pain, decreased signs or symptoms of pregnancy
What is the most common method of surgical evacuation of uterine contents in the first and second trimesters?	First trimester: dilation and curettage (D&C); Second trimester: dilation and evacuation

Antepartum and Intrapartum Hemorrhage

Half of all third trimester bleeding is caused by what two conditions?	Placental abruption and placenta previa
What is a rare but important cause of third trimester bleeding involving the fetus?	Vasa previa
Define **placental abruption**	Premature separation of normally implanted placenta
Name eight risk factors for placental abruption.	1. HTN 2. ↑ maternal age 3. Multiparity 4. African American 5. Preterm premature rupture of membranes (PPROM) 6. Smoking tobacco 7. Cocaine use 8. Trauma
What are the signs and symptoms of placental abruption?	PAINFUL bleeding, contractions, and fetal distress/death
How is placental abruption diagnosed?	Clinically; there is a high suspicion if placenta previa is ruled out by U/S
How is placental abruption managed?	Hemodynamic support, RhoGAM if appropriate, hospitalization; bed rest if preterm; induction of mature fetus or c/s if unstable fetus or mother
What are four complications of placental abruption?	1. Hypovolemic shock 2. Disseminated intravascular coagulation (DIC) 3. Preterm delivery 4. Fetal death
Define **placenta previa**	Implantation of placenta over cervical os (total, partial, or marginal)
Name four risk factors for placenta previa.	1. h/o c/s 2. Age >35 y/o 3. Multiparity 4. Smoking
What is the most common sign of placenta previa?	PAINLESS bleeding
How is placenta previa diagnosed?	Ultrasound

How is placenta previa managed?	Hemodynamic support, RhoGAM if appropriate, expectant management; delivery by c/s if fetus is mature or if patient is unstable
Name four complications of placenta previa.	1. Hypovolemic shock 2. Preterm delivery 3. ↑ fetal anomalies (2×) 4. Placenta accreta
Define *placenta accreta* and its variants, *increta* and *percreta*.	*Accreta*—placenta abnormally Attaches to myometrium; *Increta*—Invades myometrium; *Percreta*—Penetrates through myometrium to serosa
What are four risk factors for placenta accreta?	1. Placenta previa 2. h/o c/s 3. h/o curettage 4. Gravida six or more
What are the signs and symptoms of placenta accreta?	Antepartum bleeding (if associated with placenta previa, otherwise asymptomatic)
How is placenta accreta diagnosed?	U/S or MRI (false positive can occur with both)
How is placenta accreta managed?	Uterine packing to stop PP bleeding or hysterectomy
Define vasa previa	Fetal vessels passing over the internal cervical os → cord compression and possibly, rupture
What is the incidence of fetal mortality if the fetal vessel ruptures?	>50%
What is a major risk factor for vasa previa?	Velamentous cord insertion with multiple gestation
What fetal tracing is associated with ruptured fetal vessel?	Sinusoidal wave (indicating fetal anemia)
What is the treatment for vasa previa?	Emergent c/s
What is a rare but devastating cause of bleeding during labor?	Uterine rupture
What are four risk factors for uterine rupture?	1. Prior c/s 2. Trauma 3. Overdistented uterus 4. Abnormal placentation

Preterm Labor (PTL)

What is PTL?	Labor before 37 weeks GA
What are eight risk factors for PTL?	1. Preterm rupture of membranes 2. h/o PTL 3. Infection 4. Multiple gestation 5. Uterine or fetal anomaly 6. Preeclampsia 7. Low socioeconomic status 8. Smoking tobacco
What are the clinical predictors of PTL?	Persistent uterine contractions, positive fetal fibronectin, ongoing cervical dilation >3 cm or effacement >80%, vaginal bleeding, and ruptured membranes
How is PTL managed?	Hydration, empiric ABX, tocolysis, and steroids if fetus 24–34 weeks GA or negative fetal lung maturity test between 34 and 37 weeks GA
Name three tocolytic agents.	$MgSO_4$, indomethacin, and terbutaline
Name three serious toxicities of $MgSO_4$.	Loss of reflexes, respiratory depression, cardiac arrest
What is the treatment for Mg toxicity?	Calcium gluconate

Premature Rupture of Membranes (PROM)

Define PROM.	Spontaneous rupture of membranes before onset of labor; if occurring preterm → PPROM
How is PROM diagnosed?	"Gush of fluid" per vagina, sterile speculum examination (avoid digital examination) to visualize dilation/ effacement; positive pool, nitrazine (alkaline blue), or ferning test
How is PROM managed?	If there are signs of chorioamnionitis (fever, ↑ WBC, maternal/fetal tachycardia, uterine tenderness) treat with antibiotics and delivery; induction of labor within 24 h of PROM if failure to progress
How is PPROM managed?	Same as PTL but without tocolysis

What is prolonged rupture of membranes?	Rupture of membranes lasting >18 h before delivery
What is the major fetal complication associated with PPROM at ≤26 weeks GA?	Pulmonary hypoplasia

Amniotic Fluid Abnormalities

What term is used to describe an amniotic fluid index (AFI) <5?	Oligohydramnios
What are the two basic mechanisms of oligohydramnios?	1. ↓ fetal urine output 2. Chronic leak through membranes
What conditions are associated with oligohydramnios?	Congenital abnormalities, ruptured membranes, uteroplacental insufficiency, HTN, DM, ACEi, or NSAID usage, postterm pregnancy, and twin-twin transfusion syndrome
What term is used to describe AFI >20?	Polyhydramnios
What are the three basic mechanisms of polyhydramnios?	1. ↑ fetal urine output 2. ↓ fetal swallowing 3. Transudation of fluid from exposed meninges (as in spina bifida)
What conditions are associated with polyhydramnios?	NTD, alimentary canal defect, hydrops, DM, and twin-twin transfusion syndrome

Rh Incompatibility

If the mother is Rh–Rh– and the father is Rh+Rh+, what percentage of their offspring will be Rh+?	100%
If the mother is Rh–Rh– and the father is Rh+Rh–, what percentage of their offspring will be Rh+?	50%
If a woman is Rh–Rh–, by what mechanism can she become anti-D (IgG) positive?	Previous pregnancy, blood transfusion, trauma in current pregnancy
What is the effect of anti-D on an Rh+ fetus?	Anti-D can cross the placenta and cause hemolysis of fetal RBCs

Name the fetal condition characterized by severe hemolytic anemia resulting in a hyperdynamic state, heart failure, diffuse edema, ascites, and pericardial effusion.

Erythroblastosis fetalis

Which patients should receive RhoGAM and why?

Rh–/Ab– women at risk for being pregnant with Rh+ fetus

Multiple Gestation

What is the term given to fetal twins resulting from fertilization of two ova?

Dizygotic (always two amnion and two chorion)

What is the term given to twins resulting from one fertilized ovum that divides into two?

Monozygotic twins

Ethnicity (especially African descent), ↑ age, ↑ parity, and FH are contributing factors to ↑ monozygotic or dizygotic twinning?

Dizygotic

For the following types of monozygotic twins, how many days after fertilization did the ovum likely divide?

Two chorion, two amnion (DiDi), two placenta

Two to three (before trophoblastic differentiation)

One chorion, two amnion (MoDi), one placenta

Three to eight

One chorion, one amnion (MoMo), one placenta

Eight to 13

Conjoined twins

Thirteen to 15 (after formation of embryonic disk)

What signs or symptoms should raise the suspicion of a multiple gestation pregnancy?

Uterus larger than dates, excess maternal weight gain, hydramnios or unexplained maternal anemia, auscultation of more than one fetal heart, h/o ovulation induction or in vitro fertilization (IVF); confirmation by U/S

What syndrome in monochorionic twins occurs when the arterial circulation of one twin is in communication with the venous circulation of the other?

Twin-to-twin transfusion syndrome

Describe the differences between the donor and recipient twin in twin-to-twin transfusion syndrome.	**Donor:** anemia, growth restriction, and oligohydramnios; **recipient:** polycythemia, hypervolemic, cardiomegaly, and congestive heart failure (CHF)
How are twins delivered?	If first twin is vertex, then TOL; otherwise c/s
What is the most common cause of postterm pregnancy?	Inaccurate dating
What two congenital abnormalities are associated with postterm pregnancy?	Anencephaly and adrenal hypoplasia

Fetal Diagnostic Testing and Monitoring

What are the indications for prenatal genetic analysis of a fetus?	Advanced maternal age (AMA), ⊕ FH or previous child with chromosomal abnormality, fetal abnormality on U/S, abnormal serum marker screening, and unexplained intrauterine growth retardation (IUGR)
What four parameters are tested in a *quad* screen?	1. MSAFP 2. Estriol 3. hCG 4. Inhibin A
Name five causes of elevated MSAFP.	1. *NTD* 2. Inaccurate dating 3. Multiple gestation 4. Fetal abdominal wall defect 5. Fetal death
What three tests are available for checking a fetal karyotype?	1. Amniocentesis 2. Chorionic villus sampling (CVS) 3. Percutaneous umbilical blood sampling (PUBS)
At what gestational age is an amniocentesis performed and what is the incidence of complications?	16–21 weeks GA; 1/200–1/300
At what gestational age is CVS performed and what is it incidence of complications?	Nine to 11 weeks GA; 0.5–1%
What is the advantage of CVS over amniocentesis?	Offers prenatal genetic diagnosis in the first trimester and allows earlier and safer pregnancy termination if desired

What is a rare fetal complication of CVS?	Limb reduction defects
In addition to karyotype, what information does a cordocentesis reveal?	Fetal hematocrit, platelet count, and fetal blood type
What two tests are commonly used to assess fetal lung maturity?	Lecithin/sphingomyelin ratio >2 and presence of phosphatidylglycerol in amniotic fluid (both obtained by amniocentesis)
What constitutes a reactive NST?	≥2 accelerations (increased HR), each ≥15 bpm above the baseline for ≥15 s, all within 20 min
What are the five parameters of a biophysical profile (BPP)?	"Test the Baby, MAN!" Tone (extension/flexion of limb), Breathing, gross Movement, AFI, NST
What is a normal BPP score?	Eight to 10

INTRAPARTUM

Normal Labor and delivery

Triage

What is the term for irregular contractions not associated with cervical dilation or effacement?	Braxton Hicks contractions or false labor
What is the term for regular uterine contractions that cause progressive cervical dilation and/or effacement?	Labor
Name three ways to confirm rupture of membranes on vaginal examination.	Positive pooling (low sensitivity), ferning test, and nitrazine test (turns blue due to increased pH)
Do blood, semen, and vaginitis cause a false positive or a false negative nitrazine test?	False positive
Name five parameters evaluated on cervical examination to produce a Bishop's score.	Dilation, effacement, station, consistency, and position
What is the most common fetal presentation?	Vertex, occiput anterior

Progression of Labor

What are the cardinal movements of labor?

Engagement, descent, flexion, internal rotation, extension, external rotation (restitution), and expulsion

Define the following stages of labor.

First stage

Onset of labor → full cervical dilation (10 cm)

First stage—latent phase

Onset of labor → ~4 cm cervical dilation

First stage—active phase

~4 cm → 10 cm (rapid dilation)

Second stage

Complete cervical dilation → delivery of infant

Third stage

Delivery of infant → delivery of placenta (should be <30 min)

What are the three signs of placental separation?

1. Rising and firming of uterus
2. Gush of blood
3. Umbilical cord lengthening

Identify the degree of laceration described below:

Involving the skin or mucosa

First degree

Involving the fascia and muscles of perineal body

Second degree

Involving the anal sphincter

Third degree

Involving the anal mucosa (exposing lumen of rectum)

Fourth degree

Intrapartum Fetal Assessment

What is the normal range of a fetal HR (FHR)?

120–160 bpm

What is the differential diagnosis for fetal bradycardia?

Fetal distress, local anesthetics, and congenital heart block (seen with maternal SLE)

What is the differential diagnosis for fetal tachycardia?

Fetal infection or arrhythmia; maternal fever, anxiety or thyrotoxicosis; terbutaline; fetal movement and stimulation

What is the definition of a reactive FHR tracing?

≥2 accelerations (↑ in HR), each ≥15 bpm above the baseline for ≥15 s, all within 20 min

Identify the following three types of
decelerations and name their etiologies:

Symmetric deceleration that begins and ends at around the same time as contractions; looks like "mirror image" of contraction	Early deceleration; due to **head compression** stimulating vagus nerve
Most common; sharp drop and return to baseline, often preceded and followed by an acceleration (*shoulders*) and occurring at any time	Variable deceleration; due to **cord compression**
Begins at the peak of a contraction and slowly returns to the baseline after the end of a contraction	Late deceleration; due to **uteroplacental insufficiency**

Which type of deceleration is most worrisome, requiring intervention if they become repetitive?	Late deceleration
Which type of deceleration is normal and requires no intervention?	Early deceleration
Which type of deceleration is abnormal and requires intervention depending on its severity?	Variable deceleration
When is a fetal scalp pH indicated?	Nonreassuring or equivocal fetal heart tracing

Provide the range of pH for the
following fetal scalp pH interpretations:

Normal	7.25–7.35
Borderline, repeat	7.20–7.25
Acidosis, deliver immediately	<7.20
Name an alternative test to fetal scalp blood sampling.	Scalp stimulation (digital stroking of fetal scalp that evokes an acceleration suggests normal scalp pH)

Abnormal Labor and Delivery

What is the term for initiating labor in a nonlaboring patient?	Induction
What are the most common indications for labor induction?	**Maternal:** Preeclampsia and DM; **fetal:** chorioamnionitis, IUGR, postterm, and hydrops

Name three methods used to promote cervical maturation (or ripening), which would improve induction results.	1. Prostaglandin gel/insert 2. Laminaria 3. Foley
Name two common methods used to induce labor.	Pitocin (oxytocin) and amniotomy
Name two complications associated with pitocin.	Uterine hyperstimulation (stop pitocin, left lateral position, O_2) and water intoxication (prevent with strict I/O management)
What term is used to describe strengthening contractions in a laboring patient?	Augmentation
Name two methods used to augment labor.	Pitocin and amniotomy
What term is used to describe difficult labor?	Dystocia
What are the "three Ps" associated with dystocia?	Abnormalities of: 1. **Power:** uterine contractility and maternal expulsive effort (poor) 2. **Passenger:** fetus (malpresentation, breech presentation, shoulder impaction, hydrocephalus) 3. **Passage:** pelvis (android and platypelloid pelvic types, uterine fibroid)
Name the following types of breeches (buttock presentation):	
Flexed hips and extended feet → feet are near fetal head	Frank (most common)
Flexed hips and one or two flexed knees → at least 1 foot near breech	Complete
One or two hips extended → at least 1 foot below breech	Footling (least common)
How is breech usually managed?	C/s
What two other methods are used to manage breech presentation?	External cephalic version or trial of vaginal delivery
Define shoulder dystocia.	Impaction of shoulder behind pubic symphysis after delivered head
What are the risk factors for shoulder dystocia?	Macrosomia, GDM, maternal obesity, and postterm delivery
What are the fetal complications of shoulder dystocia?	Fracture of humerus/clavicle, brachial plexus injury (Erb's palsy), hypoxia, death

**Name the following maneuvers
that can help displace the shoulder
impaction:**

Pressure on maternal abdomen behind pubic symphysis	Suprapubic pressure
Sharp flexion of maternal hips	McRoberts maneuver
Pressure on posterior shoulder, rotating it in corkscrew fashion	Woods corkscrew maneuver
Pressure on accessible shoulder, pushing it toward anterior chest and decreasing shoulder-shoulder diameter	Rubin maneuver
Sweep posterior shoulder across chest, delivering arm, and rotate shoulder girdle to oblique diameter of pelvis	Delivery of posterior shoulder
Fracture of clavicle	Fracture of clavicle (last resort)
Replace infant's head back in pelvis and perform c/s	Zavanelli maneuver (last resort)

**What are the four most common
indications for c/s?**

1. Prior c/s
2. Labor dystocia
3. Fetal distress
4. Breech presentation

**Women with what kind of prior uterine
incision are candidates for vaginal
birth after cesarean (VBAC)
trial of labor (TOL)?**

Low transverse, low vertical

**What is the major complication
associated with VBAC?**

Uterine rupture

POSTPARTUM (PP)

Complications

**What is the definition of PP
hemorrhage?**

Loss of ≥500 cc blood after
completion of third stage of labor

**What are the three most common
causes of PP hemorrhage?**

1. Uterine atony
2. Retained placenta
3. Cervical/vaginal laceration

**What are the risk factors for uterine
atony?**

Uterine overdistension (multiple
gestation, hydramnios, macrosomia),
multiparity, general anesthesia, and
h/o PP hemorrhage

Describe the management of PP hemorrhage.	Uterine massage → oxytocin, methergine, or prostaglandin → explore uterus for retained placenta and explore cervix and vagina for lacerations → surgical intervention
What are three symptoms of PP endometritis?	1. Fever ≥38°C (100.4°F) within 36 h of delivery 2. Uterine tenderness 3. Malodorous lochi
What are six risk factors for PP endometritis?	1. Delivery by c/s 2. Low socioeconomic status 3. Young age 4. Prolonged ruptured membranes 5. Bacterial colonization of lower genital tract 6. Steroids
What is the treatment for PP endometritis?	Broad-spectrum ABX until afebrile for 24 h
What kind of contraception is appropriate when a mother is breastfeeding?	Progestin-only pills or Depo-Provera (less likely to ↓ milk production)

Name the following PP psychologic reactions:

Mild to suicidal depression that begins at ~4 weeks PP and can last up to 1 year PP	PP depression (may affect up to 20% of PP mothers)
Transient symptoms of depression that usually resolve by PP day 10	Maternity/PP blues (may affect up to 70% of PP mothers)

GYNECOLOGY

Benign Gynecology

Menstruation

Describe the endocrine changes that occur during each of the following phases of menstruation:

Follicular phase (proliferative, days 1–14)	1. Follicle stimulating hormone (FSH) → follicular development 2. Estrogen → endometrial proliferation and then FSH suppression 3. Progesterone low

Ovulation (day 15)

Estrogen-induced leuteinizing
hormone (LH) surge → ovulation

Luteal phase (secretory, days 15–28)

1. Corpus luteum secrete
   progesterone → endometrium
   maturation
2. ↓ LH and FSH
3. Corpus luteum regress →
   ↓ progesterone and estrogen

**What condition is characterized by
painful cramping in the lower abdomen,
with sweating, N/V, and HA—all
occurring just before or during menses?**

Dysmenorrhea

**What is the treatment for primary
dysmenorrhea?**

NSAIDs, oral contraceptive pills
(OCP)

**What is the treatment for secondary
dysmenorrhea?**

Treat underlying disease
(endometriosis, PID, ovarian cyst,
fibroids)

**What is the term for somatic and
psychologic symptoms that occur in the
second half of the menstrual cycle,
interfere with work and personal
relationships, and are followed by
symptom-free periods?**

Premenstrual dysphoric disorder
(PMDD)

**Name some characteristic physical
symptoms of PMDD.**

Bloating, breast pain, skin disorders,
HA, pelvic pain, N/V, edema,
and cravings

**Name some characteristic psychologic
symptoms of PMDD.**

Irritability, aggression, tension,
anxiety, sadness, mood lability,
and depression

**Name five treatment options for the
symptoms of PMDD.**

1. Diet and exercise
2. Selective serotonin reuptake
   inhibitor (SSRI)
3. Diuretic for edema
4. OCPs
5. Support bra for breast pain
6. Reassurance

Abnormal Uterine Bleeding

**Name the term used to describe the
following types of abnormal uterine
bleeding:**

**Heavy (>80 cc) or prolonged (>7 days)
occurring at normal intervals**

Menorrhagia

Irregular menstrual bleeding	Metrorrhagia
Frequent periods	Polymenorrhea
Menses >35 days apart	Oligomenorrhea
Absence of menstrual bleeding	Amenorrhea (pregnancy is most common cause)
What is the workup for abnormal uterine bleeding?	1. Exclude pregnancy 2. Rule out structural etiology 3. Consider dysfunctional uterine bleeding, such as anovulatory source
What is the differential diagnosis for menorrhagia and metrorrhagia?	"LACCE" Leiomyoma Adenomyosis Cervical cancer Coagulopathy Endometrial hyperplasia, or endometriosis, polyps, cancer

Contraception/Sterilization

What is the general mechanism of action (MOA) of OCP?	Ovulation suppression. **Estrogen:** inhibits FSH → prevents selection and maturation of dominant follicle; **progestin:** inhibits LH → prevents ovulation
What are three other MOAs of both combination and progestin-only formulations?	1. Thicken cervical mucus 2. ↓ fallopian tube motility 3. Cause endometrial atrophy
What are the *advantages* of OCPs?	<1% failure rate, usually ↓ cramping, protect against ovarian and endometrial cancer, ↓ PID and ectopic pregnancies, ↓ bone loss, and cause lighter menstrual flow
What are the *disadvantages* of OCPs?	Daily pill, no protection against STDs, **Side effects:** ↑ risk of irregular bleeding, nausea, irritability, amenorrhea, and breast tenderness; thrombosis, myocardial infarction (MI), cerebrovascular accident (CVA), and gallstones

What are the *contraindications* to OCPs?	Pregnancy, h/o thromboembolic d/o or stroke, chronic liver disease, undiagnosed uterine bleeding, breast cancer/carcinoma (CA), endometrial CA, smoking in women >35 y/o
How many hours after intercourse must OCPs be taken to act as emergency contraception?	Within 72 h (repeat in 12 h)
What are the *advantages* of progestin-only pills (*mini-pills*)?	Ideal for nursing mothers and women who cannot take estrogen for medical reasons
What are the *disadvantages* of progestin-only pills?	Higher failure rate (3–6%), strict compliance necessary (must take pill same time everyday)
What slow releasing, IM injection of progesterone is given every 3 months for contraception?	Depo-Provera
What are the side effects of Depo-Provera?	Irregular bleeding, conception delayed 9 months following last injection, HA, and weight gain
How do IUDs prevent pregnancy?	Elicit sterile inflammatory reaction → hostile environment for ova and sperm → inhibiting implantation
What are the complications of IUD use?	Abnormal bleeding, PID, uterine perforation, ectopic pregnancy, IUD expulsion, and failure

Menopause

What is the definition of menopause?	No menses for >1 year
What is the mean age of menopause in the United States?	51 y/o
What are the signs and symptoms of perimenopause and menopause?	Hot flashes, irritability, insomnia, depression, memory loss, dyspareunia, urinary urgency, vaginal atrophy, and ↓ bone mass
How is menopause diagnosed?	Based on history, ↑ FSH, and ↓ estradiol
Name the three indications for hormone replacement therapy (HRT).	1. Treatment of vasomotor symptoms 2. Prevention of osteoporosis (raloxifene a better choice) 3. Relief of genitourinary symptoms (topical estrogens preferred)

What are five *contraindications* to HRT?	1. Uterine bleeding of unknown origin 2. Liver disease 3. h/o DVT or PE 4. h/o breast CA 5. h/o endometrial CA
Based on the Women's Health Initiative, HRT is no longer indicated to prevent what disease?	Coronary heart disease

Infections

What age group has the highest incidence of PID in the United States?	Fifteen to 25 y/o
Aside from age what are the other risk factors for PID?	Multiple sexual partners, new sexual partner, unprotected intercourse, h/o STD, and h/o invasive gynecologic procedures
Name two organisms that cause the majority of PID cases.	*Neisseria gonorrhoeae* and *Chlamydia trachomatis* (*Escherichia coli* and *Bacteroides* cause most of the remainder of cases)
What signs are likely to be found on PE in PID?	Abdominal tenderness, adnexal tenderness, elevated temperature, and cervical motion tenderness (*chandelier sign*)
What is the differential diagnosis for *acute* pelvic pain?	"A ROPE"—**A**ppendicitis, **R**uptured ovarian cyst, **O**varian torsion/abscess, **P**ID, **E**ctopic pregnancy
What are the criteria for hospitalization in PID?	Pregnancy, peritonitis, N/V, or abscess (tuboovarian or pelvic)
What is the treatment of PID?	Broad-spectrum cephalosporin and doxycycline (*Chlamydia* coverage)
What condition presents with right upper quadrant (RUQ) pain, fever, N/V, and a significant h/o PID?	Fitz-Hugh-Curtis syndrome
Name the cause of vaginitis and appropriate treatment in each of the following clinical scenarios:	
Positive whiff test and clue cells on wet prep	Bacterial vaginosis **Tx:** Metronidazole
Pruritis and erythema, white discharge, pseudohyphae in 10% KOH	*Candida* → azole **Tx:** Antifungals

Pruritis, frothy discharge, motile and flagellated organisms on wet prep, "strawberry cervix"

Trichomonas → Metronidazole (must treat partner)

Tx: Metronidazole

What is the treatment for a Bartholin's gland abscess?

Incision and drainage (I&D), Word catheter for drainage, warm sitz baths; marsupialization for refractory disease

Endometriosis/Adenomyosis

What disorder is characterized by the growth of functional endometrial glands and stroma outside of the uterus?

Endometriosis

What is the typical parity and age of a patient with endometriosis?

Nulliparous females in twenties and thirties

Where is endometriosis most commonly found?

Uterosacral ligaments, cul-de-sac, ovaries, fallopian tubes, cervix, and colon (rarely in lungs, bladder, kidney, spine, arms, and legs)

Name two classic symptoms of endometriosis.

Cyclic pelvic pain (lesions stimulated by estrogen) and dyspareunia

Name three classic signs of endometriosis.

Fixed retroverted uterus (by adhesions), nodularity of uterosacral ligaments and cul-de-sac, and tender ovarian masses

What is the differential diagnosis for *chronic* pelvic pain?

Irritable bowel syndrome, interstitial cystitis, fibromyalgia, degenerating myomas, primary dysmenorrhea, depression, and prior psychiatric abuse

How is the diagnosis of endometriosis confirmed?

Laparoscopic visualization and biopsy

What is the term for the classic lesion filled with dark, old blood and found on the ovary in patients with endometriitis?

Chocolate cyst (endometrioma)

What is the term for old, end-stage endometriotic lesions?

Black or powder burn

What are three medical treatment options for endometriosis?

1. OCP
2. Gonadotropin-releasing hormone (GnRH) agonist (Lupron)
3. Androgen agonist (Danazol)

What are the surgical procedures for the treatment of endometriosis?	Lysis of adhesions and excision of endometriomas for those who want to preserve fertility; total hysterectomy and bilateral salpingo-oophorectomy (TAHBSO) for severe disease
What term describes the condition in which endometrial tissue is found within the myometrium?	Adenomyosis
Adenomyosis peaks in which decades?	Forties and fifties (commonly in multiparous females)
What is the triad of symptoms in adenomyosis?	1. Dysmenorrhea (noncyclic) 2. Menorrhagia 3. Enlarged uterus
What is the differential diagnosis of adenomyosis?	Myomas, dysfunctional uterine bleeding, and pregnancy with bleeding
What is the definitive method of diagnosis and ultimate treatment of adenomyosis?	Hysterectomy

Leiomyoma/Leiomyosarcoma

What is the most common pelvic tumor?	Leiomyoma (myoma/fibroid) = benign neoplasm of smooth muscle
What is the prevalence of leiomyomas in White and Black women?	Found in 25% of White women and 50% of Black women (usually of reproductive age)
Name five types of degenerations a leiomyoma may undergo once it outgrows its blood supply.	1. Hyaline 2. Myxomatous 3. Calcific 4. Red (painful hemorrhage often with pregnancy) 5. Cystic
What symptoms are associated with leiomyoma?	Abnormal uterine bleeding and pelvic pressure (majority, however, are asymptomatic)
How are leiomyomas diagnosed?	Usually by bimanual pelvic examination; imaging: U/S, abdominal x-ray (concentric calcifications), CT and MRI (rarely necessary)

What are the surgical options for unremitting, symptomatic leiomyomas?	Myomectomy for patients who wish to preserve fertility, otherwise hysterectomy

Ovarian Cyst

What is the most common type of functional ovarian cyst?	Follicular cyst (usually asymptomatic)
What type of ovarian cyst develops bilaterally in response to elevated hCG levels?	Theca lutein cyst
How are ovarian cysts diagnosed?	Pelvic examination and U/S
What is the differential diagnosis for an adnexal mass?	Ovarian cyst, ectopic pregnancy, ovarian torsion, tuboovarian abscess (TOA), endometrioma, fibroid, and ovarian neoplasm

Pelvic Mass

What is the most likely diagnosis for a pelvic mass associated with the following findings?

Painless, heavy uterine bleeding	Leiomyoma
Amenorrhea	Pregnancy
Dysmenorrhea	Endometriosis, adenomyosis, ectopic pregnancy, corpus luteum with endometrioma
Postmenopausal	Ovarian cancer
Significant h/o PID	TOA

GYNECOLOGY ONCOLOGY

Vulvar Dysplasia and Cancer (CA)

What are the signs and symptoms of vulvar cancer?	Pruritis, raised white lesion, ulceration, exophytic mass, and bleeding (most are asymptomatic)
How is vulvar cancer diagnosed?	Biopsy any suspicious lesion
What is the most common histologic type of vulvar cancer?	Squamous cell carcinoma

Cervical Dysplasia and Cancer

What are the risk factors for cervical dysplasia and cervical cancer?	Human papillomavirus (HPV) infection (especially types 16, 18, 31, 33), early intercourse, multiple sex partners, low socioeconomic status, cigarette smoking, and HIV
What is the most important screening tool for cervical dysplasia and cancer?	Pap smear
What are the guidelines for performing routine Pap smears?	Start annual Pap smear on every woman >21 y/o or within 3 years of onset of sexual activity
What are two indications for colposcopy?	High grade intraepithelial lesion (HGSIL) and any other suspicious lesion
What are the four indications for cone biopsy/ loop electrosurgical excision procedure (LEEP)?	1. Inadequate view of transformation zone on colposcopy 2. Abnormal endocervical curettage (ECC) 3. ±2 grade discrepancy between colposcopy and Pap 4. Treatment for HGSIL and lesions suspicious for microinvasion
What are the two major types of cervical cancers?	Squamous cell carcinoma (90%) and adenocarcinoma (including clear cell carcinoma from DES exposure)
What are five symptoms of cervical cancer?	1. Postcoital bleeding 2. Irregular bleeding 3. Lower extremity edema 4. Renal failure 5. Pelvic pain/pressure
Which cancer is the only gynecologic cancer that is staged clinically and not surgically?	Cervical cancer
Describe the general anatomic spread of cervical cancer in each of the following stages:	
Stage 0	Cervical intraepithelial neoplasia (CIN)
Stage I	Confined to cervix
Stage II	Extend beyond cervix but not to pelvic wall, involve upper two-thirds of vagina

Stage III	Extend to pelvic wall, involve lower one-third of vagina
Stage IV	Extend beyond pelvis, involve bladder or colon mucosa
What is the treatment for Stage I cervical cancer?	Radical hysterectomy with lymph node dissection or radiation therapy

Endometrial Hyperplasia and Cancer

What are six major risk factors for endometrial hyperplasia and endometrial cancer?	Unopposed estrogen exposure: 1. Obesity 2. Nulliparity 3. Late menopause >55 y/o 4. Chronic anovulation 5. Polycystic ovarian syndrome (PCOS) 6. Tamoxifen
What is the typical presentation of endometrial hyperplasia?	Abnormal uterine bleeding or oligomenorrhea
How is endometrial hyperplasia diagnosed?	Endometrial biopsy or D&C
What is the treatment for endometrial hyperplasia?	Progestin therapy for simple, complex, and atypical simple hyperplasia; TAHBSO for atypical complex hyperplasia
What is the most common gynecologic cancer in the United States?	Endometrial cancer
What is the most common symptom of endometrial cancer?	Postmenopausal bleeding (>90%)
What is the differential diagnosis for postmenopausal bleeding?	Endometrial hyperplasia or cancer, uterine/cervical polyp, exogenous estrogens, cervical ca, and atrophic vaginitis (if older patient, must rule out malignancy)
How is endometrial cancer diagnosed?	Endometrial biopsy
What are three general components of treatment for endometrial cancer?	Surgical staging and postoperative radiation. Progestin for recurrent disease
What four surgical procedures are involved in the staging of endometrial cancer?	1. Explanatory laparotomy 2. TAHBSO 3. Pelvic washing (cytology) 4. Pelvic and aortic lymph node dissection

Ovarian Cancer

Which gynecologic cancer has the highest mortality rate?	Ovarian cancer (usually diagnosed at Stage III or IV)
What are the three basic histologic types of ovarian cancers?	1. Epithelial 2. Germ cell 3. Sex cord stromal

Epithelial

Epithelial ovarian cancer accounts for what percentage of ovarian malignancies?	90%
What are the risk factors for ovarian cancer?	Advanced age, Caucasian race, obesity, nulliparity, and FH
What are the protective factors for ovarian cancer?	Breastfeeding, OCP, tubal ligation, hysterectomy, and multiparity
What are the early and late stage signs of ovarian cancer?	Early: Asymptomatic. Late: Pelvic mass, fluid wave, bowel obstruction
What are the three goals of surgery in epithelial ovarian cancer?	1. Establish diagnosis 2. Stage (extent of disease) 3. Debulk all visible disease if advanced cancer (include TAHBSO and nodes)
Name two adjuvant chemotherapies for epithelial ovarian cancer.	Taxol and cisplatin

Nonepithelial

What two histologic types comprise the nonepithelial tumors?	1. Germ cell tumors (GCT) 2. Sex cord-stromal tumors
What percent of GCTs are benign?	95%
In what age group are GCTs usually diagnosed?	Teens and twenties
GCTs arise from what kind of cells?	Totipotential germ cells
What are the signs and symptoms of GCTs?	May grow rapidly → pain from distension, torsion, or hemorrhage; adnexal mass, ascites, and pleural effusion
Describe the general anatomic spread of ovarian cancer in each of the following stages:	
Stage I	Limited to ovaries
Stage II	Extension from ovaries to pelvis

| Stage III | Extension to abdominal cavity |
| Stage IV | Distant metastatic disease |

Name the type of GCTs characterized by each of the following statements:

Most common malignant GCT; may be bilateral; ↑ LDH; excellent prognosis	Dysgerminoma
Yolk sac tumor; Schiller-Duval bodies; ↑ AFP; poor prognosis	Endodermal sinus tumor
Comprise 30% of all ovarian neoplasms; benign cystic teratoma; struma ovarii; and carcinoid syndrome; derived from embryonic tissue	Mature teratoma
Calcifications (like benign teratoma); cells from all three germ layers; excellent prognosis in early stages	Immature teratoma
Rare; usually diagnosed at <20 y/o; ↑ βhCG	Choriocarcinoma

Name the type of sex cord-stromal tumor characterized below:

| Estrogen secretion → precocious puberty; endometrial hyperplasia; Call-Exner bodies; inhibin tumor marker | Granulosa-theca cell tumor |
| Testosterone secretion → virilization; hirsutism; testosterone tumor marker | Sertoli-Leydig cell tumor |

| What syndrome is characterized by the triad of ovarian tumor, ascites, and right hydrothorax? | Meig's syndrome |

Gestational Trophoblastic Neoplasm (GTN)

| What is GTN? | Rare neoplasms derived from abnormal proliferation of placental tissue |

Identify the following three types of hydatidiform moles (molar pregnancies):

| Sperm fertilizes an ovum that lacks DNA; karyotype of product is 46XX (paternal DNA duplicates), no fetal parts, often signs of hyperemesis gravidarum, hyperthyroidism (rare) | Complete mole |

Two sperms fertilize normal ovum, karyotype of product is 69XXY, fetal parts present	Incomplete mole
Benign GTN that has become malignant, penetrates myometrium, rarely metastasizes	Invasive mole
What are the signs and symptoms consistent with molar pregnancy?	Passage of grape-like vesicles, new-onset HTN <20 weeks GA,
What diagnostic abnormalities are typical of molar pregnancy?	hCG >100,000; absence of fetal heart sounds; "snowstorm" on U/S
What are the four major components of the management of a molar pregnancy?	D&C to evacuate and terminate pregnancy, follow-up with weekly hCG, CXR and LFTs to check for metastasis
What malignant gestational trophoblastic tumor may occur with or after pregnancy (including ectopic, molar, or abortion)?	Choriocarcinoma
What is the characteristic histopathology of choriocarcinoma and how does it spread?	Invasive sheets of trophoblasts associated with hemorrhage and necrosis; metastasizes hematogenously
What is the treatment for choriocarcinoma?	Chemotherapy (almost 100% remission if nonmetastatic)

REPRODUCTIVE ENDOCRINOLOGY

Infertility

What is the definition of infertility?	Inability to conceive after 12 months of unprotected sexual intercourse
What is the incidence of infertility among couples?	15%
What are four major categories of infertility?	Male factor (30%), ovulatory defect (30%), tubal factor (30%), unknown/other factors (10%)
What is a normal sperm count in semen analysis?	≥20 million/mL

What are three methods used to establish ovulation?	1. Basal body temperature: should ↑ by 0.5°C after ovulation occurs 2. Progesterone: 4 ng/mL in luteal phase confirm ovulation 3. Endometrial biopsy: Should see secretory phase
How are the uterus and fallopian tubes evaluated in the workup of female factor infertility?	Hysterosalpingography: Look for obstruction → if negative → exploratory laparoscopy: look for adhesions, endometriosis
What is the treatment of infertility caused by anovulation?	Clomiphene or FSH

Dysfunctional Uterine Bleeding

Define dysfunctional uterine bleeding.	Anovulatory, abnormal uterine bleeding due to hormonal disruption and not due to organic cause (e.g., polyps/cervicitis)
How is dysfunctional uterine bleeding diagnosed?	Diagnosis of exclusion; must rule out organic lesions of reproductive tract, iatrogenic causes, gestational disorders, and coagulopathies
Name two common situations in which dysfunctional uterine bleeding may occur.	1. Extremes of reproductive life: Adolescents who have not yet established regular cycles and perimenopausal women 2. After changes in lifestyle: Factors such as diet and stress can cause regular cycles to become irregular

Amenorrhea

What is the definition of primary (1°) amenorrhea?	Absence of menses by age 16
What are the Müllerian structures?	Fallopian tubes, uterus, and upper one-third of vagina (not ovaries)
What are three general causes of 1° amenorrhea?	1. Outflow tract obstruction 2. Ovarian failure 3. Hypothalamic disorder
If the uterus is absent, what test should be ordered in the workup of 1° amenorrhea?	Karyotype
What is the definition of 2° amenorrhea?	Absence of menses ≥6 months in a woman with h/o normal menses

What is the most common cause of 2° amenorrhea?	Pregnancy

Name the cause of 2° amenorrhea described below:

Uterine scarring, adhesions from D&C, c/s, or myomectomy	Asherman syndrome
Surgical or obstetrical trauma	Cervical stenosis
Pan-hypopituitarism resulting from pituitary infarction caused by PP shock or hemorrhage	Sheehan's syndrome
↑ prolactin production	Prolactinoma
Idiopathic or due to wedge resection of ovary	Premature ovarian failure
Excessive exercising	Hypothalamic etiology
↓ T3/T4 → ↑ thyrotropin-releasing hormone (TRH) and prolactin	Hypothyroidism
Chronic anovulation, ↑ LH/FSH ratio; triad of amenorrhea, hirsutism, and obesity	Polycystic ovarian syndrome (PCOS)
Side effect of antipsychotic medications	Drug-induced hyperprolactinemia
Patients with PCOS are at risk for what three conditions?	1. Infertility 2. DM 3. Endometrial hyperplasia/CA

Provide the treatment for the following causes of amenorrhea:

Hypothalamic	Tumor removal, weight gain, stress relief, and exogenous GnRH
Pituitary	Tumor removal, bromocriptine (prolactin inhibitor), and exogenous FSH/LH
Ovarian	**PCOS:** Clomiphene for fertility, progestin-containing contraception to prevent endometrial hyperplasia, and weight loss to prevent DM; **Ovarian failure:** OCPs, donor egg
Uterine	Surgery for lysis of adhesions

UROGYNECOLOGY

Pelvic Prolapse

Name four types of pelvic prolapses	1. Cystocele 2. Rectocele 3. Enterocele 4. Uterine prolapse
What are the risk factors for pelvic organ prolapse?	Childbirth injury, aging, estrogen deficiency, connective tissue weakness, constipation, obesity, and coughing
What are the signs and symptoms of pelvic organ prolapse?	Pressure, organ protrusion, incontinence, dyspareunia, groin pain
How is pelvic organ prolapse diagnosed?	Manual inspection of urethra, vagina, perineum, and anal sphincter
What are nonsurgical management options for pelvic organ prolapse?	Lifestyle changes: stop smoking, lose weight, Kegel exercises, prevent constipation; pessary: intravaginal device to support prolapse
When is surgical treatment a good option for pelvic organ prolapse?	Symptomatic prolapse refractory to pessary

Urinary Incontinence

Provide the name and treatment for each type of incontinence described below:	
Bladder pressure → urethral pressure due to increased abdominal pressure from coughing, sneezing, running	Stress incontinence (usually due to urethral hypermobility ± sphincter dysfunction) **Tx:** Kegel exercises, estrogen therapy, alpha-adrenergic drugs, surgery (Burch, transvaginal tape [TVT])
Overactivity of bladder smooth muscle	Detrusor instability *or* urge incontinence (may be due to neurologic disease or irritation) **Tx:** Anticholinergics and timed voiding

Overdistension of bladder	Overflow incontinence **Tx:** Alpha adrenergics, striated muscle relaxants, and self-catheterization

MAKE THE DIAGNOSIS

40 y/o G4P5 female who just delivered twins followed by two whole placentas now has copious vaginal bleeding; PE: ~800 cc blood in 5 min, boggy uterus	Uterine atony
60 y/o postmenopausal, nulliparous, obese female with 5-year h/o HRT presents with vaginal spotting; PE: normal pelvic examination; workup (W/U): abnormal endometrial biopsy	Endometrial cancer
39 y/o G2P1 Black female at 28 weeks gestation presents with increasing left lower quadrant (LLQ) tenderness; PE: abdominal tenderness, asymmetric uterine shape; U/S: 5 cm × 7 cm uterine mass	Submucosal leiomyoma (with red degeneration)
45 y/o female with recent h/o hysterectomy now presents with constant urinary leakage; PE: clear fluid in vaginal vault; W/U: clear fluid Cr = 15 ⊕ methylene blue test	Vesicovaginal fistula
30 y/o G1P0 obese female at 32 weeks gestation (verified by LMP) presents for her first prenatal visit; PE: fundal height = 37 cm, FHT are within normal limits (WNL); U/S: AFI = 27 with single intrauterine pregnancy; glucola = 210 mg/dL	Gestational diabetes mellitus (GDM)
23 y/o G1P0 female at 12 weeks gestation presents with vaginal spotting and N/V; PE: 3 cm cervical dilation, U/S: intrauterine pregnancy with cardiac activity	Inevitable abortion
25 y/o G1P1 female who just delivered a 3500 g baby continues to have vaginal bleeding after delivery of placenta; PE: vaginal laceration dissecting the perineum with an intact anal sphincter	Second degree laceration

23 y/o nulligravid female with multiple partners presents with abdominal tenderness and fever; PE: cervical motion tenderness, uterine tenderness, no adnexal tenderness, no genital lesions; U/S: uterus and adnexae are WNL	Pelvic inflammatory disease (PID)
32 y/o G2P1 female at 37 weeks gestation presents in labor; PE: active phase of first stage of labor; W/U: FHR = 130 s, tracing shows shallow symmetrical decelerations in the "mirror image" of each contraction	Fetal head compression
42 y/o G2P1 Asian female at 10 weeks gestation presents with N/V; PE: ↑ HR, ↑ BP, closed cervical os; W/U: βhCG = 10,000; U/S shows "snowstorm" pattern and no IUP; karyotype: 46XX	Complete molar pregnancy
18 y/o sexually active female presents for annual gynecologic examination; PE: red and tender cervix, no uterine or adnexal tenderness; W/U: no growth on culture	Cervicitis from *Chlamydia* infection
68 y/o Caucasian female with h/o ovarian cancer, surgical staging, and taxol/carboplatin therapy 2 years ago, now presents with bloating; PE: ascites and weight loss; W/U: CA-125 = 1200	Recurrent ovarian cancer
19 y/o G1P0 Black female with twin gestation at 35 weeks gestation presents with headaches and blurred vision; PE: BP = 148/102, facial edema, no abdominal tenderness or hyperreflexia; W/U: 2+ protein on urine dipstick	Mild preeclampsia
28 y/o G3P2 female presents at term in labor; PE: fetal head at top of fundus by Leopold's maneuvers; U/S: breech presentation with both feet near fetal head	Frank breech
30 y/o G2P1 female at 34 weeks gestation presented with PTL and has been on $MgSO_4$ for 24 h; PE: lethargy, ↓↓ DTRs; W/U: ECG shows ↑ PR and QT intervals	Magnesium toxicity (>10 meq/L)
17 y/o G1P1 single female who is 7 months PP now presents with 6-month h/o weight loss, insomnia, and dysphoria; PE: poor attention to personal appearance; W/U: TFTs are WNL	Post-partum depression

31 y/o nulligravid female with h/o infrequent menses and Type 2 DM presents with infertility; PE: obese, facial hair, female phenotype; W/U: LH:FSH ratio > 3; progesterone challenge test induces menses

Polycystic ovarian syndrome (PCOS)

18 y/o G1P0 female at 22 weeks gestation presents with persistent N/V; PE: poor skin turgor, dry mucous membranes; W/U: hypochloremic alkalosis; TFT, LFTs, amylase, and lipase are all WNL

Hyperemesis gravidarum

37 y/o G2P1 Black female at 34 weeks gestation who smokes $1/2$ ppd presents with painful vaginal bleeding and contractions; PE: ↑ HR, uterine tenderness, blood in vaginal vault

Placental abruption

65 y/o G4P4 female with h/o chronic bronchitis presents with urinary incontinence when coughing or laughing, but denies nocturia; PE: incontinence when asked to cough, cotton swab test = 45°; UA and culture are WNL

Stress incontinence

24 y/o G1P0 female at 28 weeks gestation presents for a routine U/S; PE: consistent with 28-week twin gestation; U/S: same-sex twins sharing one placenta, with polyhydramnios of one amniotic sac and oligohydramnios of the other; fetal weight difference >20%

Twin-to-twin transfusion syndrome

21 y/o female with h/o PID presents with cramping and vaginal spotting; PE: abdominal tenderness; W/U: ⊕ βhCG; U/S: empty uterus

Ectopic pregnancy

23 y/o G2P2 female with h/o uncontrolled Type 1 DM presents 1 day after c/s with fever; PE: fever=102°, uterine tenderness, and malodorous lochi; W/U: WBC=16,000; UA and urine culture are negative

Endometritis

39 y/o G2P1 female at 18 weeks gestation presents for routine prenatal care visit; PE: consistent with 18 wk pregnancy; W/U: Triple Screen shows ↓ AFP and estriol, and ↑ βhCG; U/S: thickened nuchal skin and short femurs

Down's syndrome fetus (increased likelihood)

30 y/o G1P0 Caucasian female at 32 weeks gestation present with malaise, N/V, and abdominal tenderness; PE: BP = 150/98, RUQ tenderness; W/U: platelets = 70,000, ↑ LFTs; Peripheral blood smear shows hemolysis	HELLP syndrome
36 y/o HIV-positive female with h/o tobacco and heroin use presents with vaginal spotting; PE: cachexia, friable cervix with a mass	Cervical cancer
27 y/o nulligravid female presents with 6-month h/o pelvic pain that increases when she is menstruating; PE: tender left ovary; U/S: 3 cm left adnexal mass; UA, cultures, and pregnancy test are all negative	Endometrioma
29 y/o G1P0 female at 31 weeks gestation presents with complaint of leaking clear fluid; she denies contractions, vaginal bleeding, or fevers; PE: sterile speculum examination shows pool of clear fluid in vaginal vault; W/U: nitrazine test is blue	Preterm premature rupture of membranes (PPROM)
61 y/o G5P5 female with h/o traumatic labor 20 years prior presents with pelvic pressure and urinary frequency; PE: cervix visualized and palpated just behind the introitus	Prolapsed uterus
19 y/o nulligravid female who presents with dyspareunia; PE: involuntary spasms preclude vaginal examination	Vaginismus
36 y/o G2P2 female with h/o abdominal hysterectomy for unrelenting postpartum hemorrhage and hypotension (8 months ago) presents with $2°$ amenorrhea since then; W/U: negative βhCG, ↓ serum prolactin	Sheehan's syndrome
24 y/o G1P0 female at 33 weeks gestation is hospitalized for polyhydramnios of unknown etiology; PE: fundal height greater than dates; W/U: fetal heart tracing shows sinusoidal wave pattern	Cord prolapse

CHAPTER 6

Pediatrics

GENETIC DEFECTS

Name the trisomy described by
the following statements:

Endocardial cushion defects, duodenal atresia, Hirschsprung's disease, hypothyroidism, mental retardation (MR), leukemia, Alzheimer's-like dementia	Trisomy 21 (Down's syndrome)
Rocker-bottom feet and micrognathia	Trisomy 18 (Edward's syndrome)
Microphthalmia, polydactyly, microcephaly, and cleft lip/palate	Trisomy 13 (Patau syndrome)
Most common chromosomal abnormality	Trisomy 21 (Down's syndrome)

What syndrome is characterized by
the karyotype 45XO?

Turner's syndrome

Name five dysmorphic features
associated with Turner 'syndrome.

1. Lymphedema of the hands and feet
2. Shield-shaped chest
3. Widely spaced nipples
4. Webbed neck
5. Low hair line

Name three common cardiac defects
associated with Turner's syndrome.

Coarctation of the aorta, bicuspid
aortic valve, and aortic stenosis

What gonadal abnormality occurs in
100% of Turner's patients?

Gonadal dysgenesis

What is the most common cause of
hypogonadism in males?

Klinefelter's syndrome (47XXY)

What are five clinical manifestations
of Klinefelter's syndrome?

1. Small phallus
2. Small testes (hypospermia)
3. Gynecomastia

	4. Increased height
	5. Learning disability with normal IQ
What is a Barr body?	An inactivated X chromosome associated with Klinefelter's syndrome
What hormone is used to treat Klinefelter's syndrome?	Testosterone (improves secondary sexual characteristics and prevents gynecomastia)
What syndrome is associated with uncontrollable appetite and Pickwickian syndrome?	Prader-Willi syndrome
What is the mode of inheritance in Prader-Willi syndrome?	Paternal imprinting
What disease is known as the "happy puppet" syndrome?	Angelman syndrome (due to ataxic gait and tiptoe walk, patients also have severe MR and episodes of uncontrollable laughter)
What is the mode of inheritance in Angelman syndrome?	Maternal imprinting
What inherited syndrome, characterized by severe MR, is caused by trinucleotide repeats?	Fragile X syndrome

DEVELOPMENT

Milestones

At what age is an average child expected to do the following:

Walk	12 months
Run	18 months
Display stranger anxiety	7 months
Use a pincer grasp	9 months (**Remember:** An upsidedown pincer grasp forms the number **9**)
Hold their head up	3 months
Sit up without support	6 months
Say their first word	12 months (**one** word at **1** year)
Use two-word combinations	24 months (**two** words at **2** years)

Use three-word sentences	36 months (**three** words at **3** years)
Crawl	9 months
List the sequence of events that occur in female puberty.	Thelarche, growth spurt, pubarche, menarche
List the sequence of events that occur in male puberty.	Testicular enlargement, penile enlargement, growth spurt, pubarche
Name the Tanner stage:	
Breast bud development and enlargement of areolar diameter.	Tanner stage II
Increased darkening of scrotal skin.	Tanner stage IV

Vaccinations

Give the appropriate timing for each of the following vaccinations:	
Hepatitis B	Birth (Hep **B** at birth), 1–4 , 6–18 months
Polio	2 months, 4 months, 6–18 months/ 4–6 years
Measles, mumps, and rubella (MMR)	>12 months, 4–6 years
Diphtheria-tetanus-pertussis (DTaP)	2 months, 4 months, 6 months, 15–18 months/4–6 years; tetanus booster required every 10 years
Haemophilus influenzae **type b (Hib)**	2, 4, 6, 12 months (not indicated in patients greater than 5 years)
Pneumococcus (PCV)	For children younger than 5 years; 2 months, 4 months, 6 months, 12–15 months
What type of polio vaccine is recommended in the United States?	Inactivated polio vaccine (IPV) (the oral vaccine [OPV] is the number one cause of polio in the United States)
What age must a child be in order to receive a varicella vaccination?	Greater than 12 months
Name the vaccination(s):	
Contraindicated in immunocompromised patients	MMR, varicella, and oral polio vaccine (OPV)
Containing egg protein	MMR and influenza

Required in asplenic patients	Pneumococcal, meningococcal, and Hib vaccines (encapsulated organism vaccines)
Contraindicated in patients with progressive neurologic disorders or encephalopathy within 7 days of administration	DTaP (the pertussis component is associated with seizures)

Failure to Thrive

Define failure to thrive (FTT).	FTT is a condition in which an infant's weight gain and growth are far below usual levels for age
List the major risk factors of FTT.	1. Low socioeconomic status 2. Low maternal age 3. Low birth weight 4. Caregiver neglect 5. Maternal or fetal disease
What are the most common organic causes of FTT?	1. Congenital heart disease 2. Cystic fibrosis (CF) 3. Celiac sprue 4. Pyloric stenosis 5. Infection 6. Gastroesophageal reflux

NEONATALOGY

What determines the Apgar score?	APGAR (0, 1, or 2 in each category) Appearance (blue/pale, pink trunk, all pink) Pulse (0, <100, >100) Grimace with stimulation (0, grimace, grimace and cough) Activity (limp, some, active) Respiratory effort (0, irregular, regular)
Determine the Apgar score:	
Newborn with a pink trunk, HR = 50, a grimace and cough when stimulated, strong muscle tone, and an irregular respiratory effort	Seven

A blue newborn, HR = 30, a grimace when stimulated, appears limp, and has no respiratory effort	Two
What serologic marker is used to detect the HIV status in an infant of a HIV ⊕ mother?	HIV DNA levels
What three organisms are the most common causes of neonatal sepsis?	"GEL" Group B streptococci, *Escherichia coli, Listeria monocytogenes*
What is the treatment regimen for a neonate with sepsis?	Ampicillin and gentamicin or ampicillin and cefotaxime for 10–14 days
What is the differential diagnosis of respiratory distress in a newborn?	Respiratory distress syndrome (RDS), meconium aspiration, transient tachypnea of the newborn, congenital pneumonia, congenital heart disease
What is the most common cause of respiratory failure in a premature newborn?	RDS
What is the pathogenesis of RDS?	Lack of adequate surfactant production causing alveolar collapse
What is the typical presentation of RDS?	Tachypnea, grunting, retractions, and nasal flaring in the first few hours of life
What is the typical course of RDS?	Progressive worsening and impending respiratory failure in the first 48–72 h of life
What are the characteristic findings on chest x-ray (XR) of RDS?	Diffuse atelectasis and a ground-glass appearance
What is the treatment of RDS?	Usually requires intubation and surfactant administration
What are the complications of chronic treatment of RDS?	Bronchopulmonary dysplasia, retinopathy of prematurity, and barotrauma from positive pressure ventilation
What is physiologic jaundice?	Transient, unconjugated hyperbilirubinemia caused by large bilirubin load that overwhelms a maturing liver system
What three features differentiate physiologic jaundice from pathologic jaundice?	1. Hyperbilirubinemia in the first 24 h of life 2. Prolonged jaundice 3. Conjugated hyperbilirubinemia

Name the fatal complication of neonatal hyperbilirubinemia.	Kernicterus (bilirubin staining of the basal ganglia, pons, and cerebellum)
Name the two therapies available for severe jaundice.	1. Phototherapy 2. Exchange transfusion
What is the pathognomonic radiographic finding in patients with necrotizing enterocolitis?	Pneumatosis intestinalis (air in the bowel wall)

Name the congenital anomaly in the described below:

Neonate with inability to feed, excessive salivation, and recurrent aspiration pneumonia with a polyhydramniotic mother	Tracheoesophageal fistula
Neonate with bilious emesis and a "double-bubble" sign on abdominal radiograph	Duodenal atresia
Neonate born with abdominal viscera herniating through the umbilicus, contained in a sac	Omphalocele (gastroschisis contains no sac)

CONGENITAL HEART DISEASE

Name the five congenitally acquired cyanotic heart lesions.	Remember: "12345" 1. Truncus arteriosus (**one** arterial vessel overrides ventricles) 2. Transposition of the great vessels (**two** arteries are switched) 3. **Tri**cuspid atresia 4. **Tetra**logy of Fallot 5. Total anomalous pulmonary venous return (**five** words)

Name the cyanotic heart lesion described below:

Most common cyanotic lesion presenting in the first 2 weeks of life	Transposition of the great vessels
"Boot-shaped heart" and decreased pulmonary vascular markings on CXR	Tetralogy of Fallot
Cardiomegaly and an "egg-shaped silhouette" on CXR	Transposition of the great vessels

Treatment consists of arterial switch performed in the first 2 weeks of life	Transposition of the great vessels (left ventricle will decompensate if procedure is delayed longer than 2 weeks)
Cardiac defect wherein pulmonary venous blood is directed to the right atrium (RA)	Total anomalous pulmonary venous return
Increased right ventricular outflow obstruction that causes cyanosis by increasing right to left shunting	Tetralogy of Fallot (*tet spells*)
What physiologic, musical murmur is often present in young children?	Still's murmur
Name the four defects in tetralogy of Fallot.	"PROVe" 1. **P**ulmonic stenosis 2. **R**ight ventricular hypertrophy 3. **O**verriding aorta 4. **V**entricular septal defect (VSD)
What congenital heart lesion is defined as tricuspid valve displacement into the right ventricle?	Ebstein anomaly
Which maternally ingested drug is associated with Ebstein anomaly?	Lithium
Name three congenital acyanotic heart lesions.	1. VSD 2. Atrial septal defect (AS**D**) 3. Patent ductus arteriosus (PDA)— all with letter "**D**"
What is the most common congenital heart defect?	Ventricular septal defect
What is the feared complication of a large, untreated VSD?	Eisenmenger syndrome
What results from a deficiency of the endocardial cushion?	Atrioventricular (AV) canal defect— ostium primum ASD and inlet VSD
What congenital infection is associated with a PDA?	Rubell-**A** → PD**A**
What is the mode of inheritance in hypertrophic cardiomyopathy?	Autosomal dominant
What is the clinical triad of hypertrophic cardiomyopathy?	Chest pain, dyspnea on exertion, and syncope (common cause of sudden cardiac death in athletes)
What are the most common causes of sinus tachycardia?	Fever, dehydration, exercise, and anemia

Name the key ECG manifestation of Wolff-Parkinson-White syndrome.	Delta wave (caused by preexcitation of the ventricle via the bypass tract)
Which antiarrhythmic drug is contraindicated in Wolff-Parkinson-White syndrome?	Digoxin (by slowing the AV node, a bypass tract can repolarize and potentially create an atrial tachyarrhythmia), use beta–blocker instead

PULMONARY

What common disease is characterized by reversible airway obstruction with accompanying bronchial hypersensitivity?	Asthma
What disease is caused by a defect in the chloride channel on epithelial cells?	CF
Name the mode of inheritance and the chromosome responsible for CF.	Autosomal recessive (AR) on chromosome 7 (CF)
What gastrointestinal (GI) manifestation in the neonate is pathognomonic for CF?	Meconium ileus (intestinal obstruction following inspissation of meconium)
What is the most common manifestation of CF in infants and children?	Failure to thrive
What is the most common bacterial cause of pneumonia in children?	*Streptococcus pneumoniae*
Name the most common clinical manifestations of CF in the following organ systems:	
Respiratory	1. Nasal polyps 2. Sinusitis 3. Bacterial pneumonia 4. Digital clubbing 5. Cough 6. Hemoptysis
GI	Pancreatic insufficiency (causing malabsorption, diarrhea, and failure to thrive), diabetes, rectal prolapse, and meconium ileus
Hepatobiliary	Neonatal jaundice, portal hypertension, and cirrhosis
Reproductive	Impaired fertility in males

Name the diagnostic test of choice in CF.	Sweat chloride test (levels greater than 60 mEq/L)
What is the recommended treatment for CF?	DNAse (Pulmozyme), pancreatic enzymes, and vitamins

INFECTIOUS DISEASE

Name the most common types of group A streptococcal infections.	Peritonsillar abscess, retropharyngeal abscess, rheumatic fever, poststreptococcal glomerulonephritis (PSGN)
Which complication is not avoided with antibiotic treatment?	PSGN
Name the four clinical manifestations of PSGN.	Hematuria, oliguria, hypertension, and edema
Name the viral exanthem associated with the following clinical manifestations:	
Cough, coryza, conjunctivitis	Measles (rubeola)
Fever with a vesicular rash at different stages	Varicella (chickenpox)
Maculopapular rash, febrile seizures, and HHV-6 infection	Roseola infantum
"Slapped cheek" appearance with parvovirus B19 infection	Erythema infectiosum (fifth disease)
Painful ulcers on the tongue and oral mucosa and a maculopapular rash on the distal limbs and buttocks	Hand, foot, and, mouth (-and butt) disease (coxsackievirus)
What is the differential diagnosis for upper airway obstruction?	Foreign body aspiration, croup, epiglottitis, retropharyngeal abscess, bacterial tracheitis, angioedema
Croup or epiglottitis?	
Most commonly caused by parainfluenza virus infection	Croup
Presents with high fever, "sniffing dog" position, toxic appearance, and drooling	Epiglottitis
Very rare due to the Hib vaccination	Epiglottitis

Responds best to racemic epinephrine	Croup
Frequently requires emergent endotracheal intubation	Epiglottitis
"Steeple sign" on anteroposterior (AP) neck films	Croup (think of a Group of people going to the steeple)
Presents with inspiratory stridor and a "barky cough"	Croup
What are the three most common organisms that cause otitis media (OM)?	*S. pneumonia*, nontypeable *H. influenza, Moraxella catarrhalis*
What does the otologic examination reveal in OM?	Bulging tympanic membrane (TM), loss of TM light reflex, decreased mobility of the TM on pneumatic otoscopy
What is the typical treatment for OM?	High-dose amoxicillin (80–90 mg/kg/day) for 10 days
What pathogen causes most cases of bronchiolitis?	Respiratory syncytial virus (RSV)
What is the recommended treatment for a neonate with meningitis?	Ampicillin and gentamicin or ampicillin and cefotaxime (older children—vancomycin and ceftriaxone)

GASTROENTEROLOGY

Name the GI disease characterized by the following descriptions:	
Most common indication for surgical intervention	Appendicitis
Most common cause of bowel obstruction in children less than 2 years of age	Intussusception
Characterized by projectile, nonbilious vomiting in first-born males less than 2 months of age	Pyloric stenosis
Air-enema is diagnostic and therapeutic	Intussusception
Physical examination reveals an olive-shaped, mobile, nontender mass	Pyloric stenosis

Manifests as crampy, abdominal pain with emesis and bloody, mucous in stool (*currant jelly* stool)	Intussusception
Presents as painless, rectal bleeding	Meckel's diverticulum
Failure of ganglionic cell migration	Hirschsprung's disease
Arises from "lead points" and is described as a "sausage-like mass" on examination	Intussusception
Diagnosis requires a technetium pertechnetate scan that detects ectopic gastric mucosa	Meckel's diverticulum
Diagnosis requires ultrasound and treatment is by surgical pylorotomy	Pyloric stenosis
Presents as bilious emesis in a child <1 month of age; diagnosed by upper GI series	Malrotation
Risk factors include Meckel's diverticulum, intestinal lymphoma, Henoch-Schönlein purpura, celiac disease, CF, and infection	Intussusception (all can act as potential *lead points*)
Describe the major characteristics of Meckel's diverticulum.	"Rule of 2s"
	Males are affected **two** times as often as females
	2 feet proximal to ileocecal valve
	2 types of ectopic mucosa (gastric or pancreatic)
	2% of population
	2 years of age

NEPHROLOGY

What is the most frequent clinical sign of vesicoureteral reflux?	Recurrent urinary tract infections (UTIs)
What is the diagnostic test of choice in vesicoureteral reflux?	Voiding cystourethrogram (VCUG)
Name the most common penile congenital anomaly.	Hypospadias
What are the two major complications of cryptorchidism?	Impaired sperm production and increased risk of malignancy

Name the four characteristics of
nephrotic syndrome.

Proteinuria, hypoalbuminemia,
hyperlipidemia, and edema

What is the most common cause of
nephrotic syndrome in children and
what is the treatment?

Minimal change disease, steroids
(best prognosis)

What is the hallmark of
glomerulonephritis?

Hematuria

Name the glomerulonephritis
characterized by the following
descriptions:

    Sudden onset of hematuria 2 weeks
    after streptococcal pharyngitis

Acute PSGN (most common)

    Hematuria with an insidious
    progression to renal failure and
    encephalopathy

Rapidly progressive
glomerulonephritis

    Palpable purpura on the lower limbs
    and buttocks followed by abdominal
    pain and hematuria

Henoch-Schönlein purpura

    Nephritic clinical picture accompanied
    by sensorineural hearing loss

Alport's syndrome

    Elevated anti-DNAse and low
    complement C3 levels

Acute PSGN

ENDOCRINOLOGY

What disease results from a lack of
insulin production by β-cells in the
pancreas?

Insulin-dependent diabetes mellitus
(type 1)

What is the typical presentation of
type 1 diabetes?

Polyuria, polydypsia, fatigue, and
abdominal pain

What three screening tests should
be performed annually in the pediatric
patient with type 1 diabetes?

Urine screening for
microalbuminemia, ophthalmologic
examination for retinopathy, and
lipid profile for hyperlipidemia

What are the key features of
diabetic ketoacidosis (DKA)?

Hyperglycemia, ketoacidosis,
dehydration, and lethargy

What are the general treatment goals
for DKA?

Fluid resuscitation, insulin therapy
(until ketoacidosis resolves), and
electrolyte management

What is the most feared complication
in the treatment of DKA?

Cerebral edema (caused by rapid
changes in serum osmotic pressure)

Constitutional delay or familial short stature?

Normal growth velocity at or below the fifth percentile	Constitutional delay
Growth curves fall below the fifth percentile with abnormal growth velocity	Familial short stature
Delay in bone age	Constitutional delay
Puberty is typically delayed	Constitutional delay
Normal bone age	Familial short stature

List the six most common pathologic causes of short stature.	1. Growth hormone deficiency 2. Primary hypothyroidism 3. Cushing's disease 4. Chronic systemic disease 5. Psychosocial deprivation 6. Turner's syndrome
What congenital hormonal deficiency can cause severe MR?	Congenital hypothyroidism
What is the most common enzyme deficiency in congenital adrenal hyperplasia?	21-hydroxylase deficiency
What are the clinical manifestations of 21-hydroxylase deficiency?	Ambiguous genitalia in females, hyponatremia and hyperkalemia (from lack of aldosterone), and hypoglycemia (from insufficient cortisol)
The elevation of what hormone is diagnostic for 21-hydroxylase deficiency?	17-hydroxyprogesterone
What hormonal therapy is used to treat 21-hydroxylase deficiency?	Cortisol (for suppression of androgen production) and mineralcorticoids (for electrolyte balance)

HEMATOLOGY

Name the cause of anemia in the following descriptions:

Most common cause of anemia in the pediatric population	Iron deficiency anemia
Patients present with bone/chest pain, dactylitis, priapism, or strokes	Sickle cell disease

Inherited hemolytic anemia caused by malformation or malfunction of globin subunits of the hemoglobin molecule	Thalassemia
Treatment of acute symptoms consists of oxygen, fluids, analgesia, antibiotics, and exchange transfusion	Sickle cell disease
Caused by exclusive feeding with cow's milk without mineral supplementation	Iron deficiency anemia (iron in breast milk is more bioavailable)
Typically presents at 4 months of age as hemoglobin F levels begin to decline	Sickle cell disease
X-linked recessive disease that presents during oxidative stress caused by fava beans or drug exposure (dapsone, sulfonamides, and antimalarials)	Glucose-6-phosphate dehydrogenase (G6PD) deficiency
Patients are at greatest risk for infection and sepsis from *H. influenza* and *S. pneumoniae*	Sickle cell disease (spleen may be compromised due to autoinfarction)

Name the complication of sickle cell disease described below:

Caused by repeated infarction of lung tissue	Acute chest syndrome
Painful swelling of the hands and feet	Dactylitis
Potentially fatal complication typically induced by parvovirus B19 infection	Aplastic crisis (must check reticulocyte count in sickle patients)
Complication that causes pain, priapism, gallbladder disease, chronic renal failure, splenic infarction and avascular necrosis of the femoral head	Vasoocclusive crisis
Sickle cells cause microvascular obstruction and lead to fibrosis of the spleen	Autoinfarction (↑ susceptibility of infection with encapsulated organisms)

Name the coagulation disorder(s) characterized by the following statements:

X-linked recessive disease caused by a deficiency in factor VIII	Hemophilia A
X-linked recessive disease caused by a deficiency in factor IX	Hemophilia B

Treated with desmopressin acetate (DDAVP)	von Willebrand's disease and hemophilia A (DDAVP causes release of factor VIII and von Willebrand's factor [vWF] from endothelial cells)
Bleeding sites are from mucous membranes, skin, and vagina during menstruation	von Willebrand's disease
Bleeding causes hemarthroses and intramuscular bleeds	Hemophilia A and B
Increase in partial thromboplastin time (PTT) with normal prothrombin time (PT) and platelet aggregation	Hemophilia A/B and von Willebrand's disease

ONCOLOGY

What is the most common childhood malignancy?	Leukemia (acute lymphocytic leukemia is the most common)
What type of leukemia is more common in African American males of any age?	AML
What type of leukemia is more common in White males, 3–5 years of age?	ALL
What is the typical initial presentation of a patient with leukemia?	Lethargy, malaise, anorexia, and weight loss
What are the typical late presenting signs of leukemia?	Bone pain and arthralgia
The cluster of petechiae, pallor, ecchymosis, and fever in a patient with a history of leukemia is evidence of what pathophysiologic process?	Bone marrow failure
What is the treatment for leukemia?	Prednisone, vincristine, and L-asparaginase
What is the most common solid tumor and the second most common malignancy in childhood?	Central nervous system (CNS) tumors
Where do CNS tumors typically occur?	Infratentorial (cerebellum, midbrain, brainstem) most adult CNS tumors are supratentorial
Name the clinical manifestations of CNS tumors.	Truncal ataxia, coordination/gait disturbances, and head tilt (due to cranial nerve palsies)

What are the symptoms of ↑ intracranial pressure (ICP)?	Headaches, vomiting, and lethargy
What are the signs of ↑ ICP?	Papilledema, altered mental status, and Cushing's triad (hypertension, bradycardia, Cheyne-Stokes respirations-a late finding)
Name the malignancy of primitive neural crest cells of the adrenal medulla and sympathetic ganglia.	Neuroblastoma
What is the most common presentation of neuroblastoma?	Painless abdominal mass
What two diagnostic tests provide the definitive diagnosis of neuroblastoma?	Elevated urinary catecholamines and pathologic identification of tumor tissue
What congenital anomalies are associated with Wilms' tumor?	**WAGR**—Wilms' tumor, Aniridia, ambiguous Genitalia, mental Retardation

Ewing's sarcoma or osteosarcoma?

Occurs on the midshaft of bones	Ewing's sarcoma (osteosarcoma at epiphysis)
Classic "sunburst appearance" on radiograph	Osteosarcoma
Malignant tumor of osteoblasts	**Osteo**sarcoma (**osteo**blasts)
Undifferentiated sarcoma	Ewing's sarcoma
↑ alkaline phosphatase may be used as a diagnostic test and as a treatment marker	Osteosarcoma
Higher probability of lung metastasis	Osteosarcoma (chest CT to rule out pulmonary metastasis)

IMMUNODEFICIENCY SYNDROMES

At what age do T-cell immunodeficiencies present and what types of infections are they characterized by?	1–3 months, broad range infections (fungal, bacterial, viral)
List two of the most common T-cell immunodeficiency syndromes.	DiGeorge's syndrome and ataxia telangiectasia

What is the embryonal deformity in DiGeorge syndrome?

Agenesis of the third and fourth pharyngeal pouch (responsible for the development of the thymus and parathyroid gland)

What are the clinical manifestations of DiGeorge syndrome?

"CATCH-22"

Cardiac anomalies (tetralogy of Fallot, interrupted aortic arch, and vascular rings)

Abnormal facies

Thymic hypoplasia

Cleft palate

Hypocalcemia

22 (chromosome 22q11 microdeletion)

Name the immunodeficiency syndrome characterized by cerebellar ataxia, oculocutaneous telangiectasia, decreased T-cell function, and low antibody levels.

Ataxia telangiectasia

At what age do B-cell deficiency syndromes typically present?

6 months (maternal antibodies protect infant up to this age)

What types of infections occur in B-cell deficiency syndromes?

Recurrent upper respiratory infections and bacteremia caused by encapsulated organisms

Name the three most common B-cell deficiency syndromes.

X-linked agammaglobulinemia, common variable immunodeficiency, and selective IgA deficiency

Name the disease characterized by a total lack of antibody production.

X-linked (Bruton's) agammaglobulinemia

Name the disease characterized by recurrent respiratory, GI, and urinary tract infections.

Selective IgA deficiency

List the two most common combined B- and T-cell immunodeficiency syndromes.

Severe combined immunodeficiency disease (SCID) and Wiskott-Aldrich syndrome

What are the clinical manifestations of Wiskott-Aldrich syndrome?

"WATER"

W—↓ IgM (W upside down)

A—↑ IgA

Thrombocytopenia

Eczema

Recurrent infections

What are the clinical manifestations of phagocytic immunodeficiency syndromes?	Poor wound healing, abscess formation, and granulomas
Name the two most common phagocytic syndromes.	Chronic granulomatous disease (X-linked recessive) and Chediak-Higashi syndrome (AR)
What chemical process is affected in patients with chronic granulomatous?	Oxidative burst that produces hydrogen peroxide
What is the defective immunologic process of Chediak-Higashi syndrome?	Neutrophil chemotaxis (may manifest as oculocutaneous albinism)

RHEUMATOLOGY

What pediatric disease is characterized by multijoint pain, fatigue, rash, lymphadenopathy, and failure to thrive?	Juvenile rheumatoid arthritis (JRA)
Name the type of JRA associated with each of the following statements:	
5+ joints, symmetric; resembles adult RA; ±rheumatoid factor (RF)	Polyarticular
Small, pink, salmon-colored macular rash; high-spiking fevers, hepatosplenomegaly (HSM)	Systemic (10–20%) "Still's disease"
<5 joints (usually weight-bearing); type 1 = females <4 y/o; type 2 = males >8 y/o	Pauciarticular (~50%)
What is the treatment for JRA?	NSAIDs and strengthening exercises; metrotrexate (MTX) = second line
What is the major ocular complication of pauciarticular JRA?	Visual loss due to iridocyclitis (routine eye examinations); typically ANA ⊕
What are the major complications of systemic JRA?	Pulmonary, hepatic, CNS, Nerve entrapment (e.g., carpal tunnel syndrome)
What laboratory value is significantly increased in patients with dermatomyositis?	Serum creatinine kinase
Name the vasculitis characterized by each of the following:	
Positive cytoplasmic antineutrophil cytoplasmic antibodies (c-ANCA)	Wegener's granulomatosis

Palpable purpura, abdominal pain, and hematuria	Henoch-Schönlein purpura
Recurrent upper and lower respiratory tract infections	Wegener's granulomatosis
Treated with IV immunoglobulin (IVIG) and high-dose aspirin	Kawasaki disease
Treated with corticosteroids and cyclophosphamide	Wegener's granulomatosis
Coronary aneurysms are the most fatal complication	Kawasaki disease
What are the clinical manifestations of Kawasaki disease?	"My HEART" My—Mucous membrane changes (fissured lips and *strawberry tongue*) Hands and extremity changes (erythema and edema) Eye changes (conjunctivitis with limbal sparing) Adenitis (painful) lymphadenitis Rash Temperature (>104°F for 5 days)

NEUROLOGY

What congenital neurologic disorder is diagnosed by an increased maternal serum alpha-fetoprotein level?	Neural tube defect
Name the perinatal supplement that can reduce the incidence of neural tube defects?	Folic acid
What type of epileptic seizure frequently presents as a blank stare in children less than 10 y/o?	Absence seizure
Name the EEG pattern that is diagnostic of absence seizures.	Three-per-second spike and wave pattern
What seizure, occurring in children between 2 and 7 months of age, manifests as extensor-flexor spasms occurring up to 100 times in a day?	Infantile spasm
Name the EEG pattern that is diagnostic of infantile spasms.	Hypsarrhythmia (chaotic pattern)

Febrile Seizures

Define febrile seizure.	Nonepileptic seizure in children 6 months to 5 years of age that occurs in the setting of fever
What is the cause of febrile seizures?	Rapidly increasing body temperature (not the absolute temperature)
Simple or complex seizure?	
Duration less than 15 min	Simple
More than one seizure in a 24-h period	Complex
Characterized by a focal seizure	Complex (simple seizures are always generalized)
Treatment consists of fever reduction (antipyretics)	Simple
Associated with a 10% risk of epilepsy	Complex (may require anticonvulsant therapy, must perform EEG and MRI to rule out neurologic disease)

Cerebral Palsy

What nonprogressive, nonhereditary movement and posture disorder is associated with perinatal brain damage?	Cerebral palsy (CP)
List the risk factors for CP.	1. Prematurity 2. MR 3. Low birth weight 4. Fetal malformation 5. Neonatal seizures 6. Neonatal cerebral hemorrhage 7. Perinatal asphyxia
What is the most frequent presenting sign of CP?	Delayed motor development (often missed until child fails to meet developmental milestones)
What percentage of CP patients show mental retardation?	About 50%
What is the most common form of CP?	Pyramidal (characterized by spasticity in all affected limbs)
What is the treatment of CP?	Benzodiazepines, dantrolene, and baclofen (goal is to reduce spasticity)

CHILD ABUSE

Name the findings in each of the
examinations listed below suggestive
of child abuse:

    Dermatologic examination

                                         Ecchymoses of varying stages
and pattern injuries (iron/cigarette
burns, immersion burns, belt
markings)

    Ocular examination

                                         Retinal hemorrhages (shaken baby
syndrome)

    X-ray examination

                                         Spiral fractures, rib fractures,
metaphyseal corner fractures;
fractures at different stages of
healing

    Genitourinary examination

                                         Sexually transmitted diseases, genital
trauma

    Head CT

                                         Subdural hematoma (shaken baby
syndrome)

MISCELLANEOUS

At what age does an average
pediatric patient triple their birth
weight?

    1 year

What two criteria must be met before
a baby can ride facing forward in
a car seat?

    Child must be 1 y/o and >20 lb

What cause of anemia occurs in
children that are strictly cow
milk-fed?

    Iron deficiency anemia (iron in breast
milk is more bioavailable)

What vitamin supplement must a child
receive that is strictly breast-fed?

    Vitamin D

What organism is associated with
hemolytic uremic syndrome?

    E. coli O157:H7

What is the differential diagnosis for
an infant with leukocoria (lack of a red
reflex)?

    Retinoblastoma, retinopathy of
prematurity, and congenital cataracts

What two classic physical examination techniques can be used to identify congenital hip dislocation?

Barlow's (posteriorsuperior hip dislocation pressure) and Ortolani's (click with hip abduction) maneuvers

Name two additional physical examination findings that suggest a congenital hip dislocation.

Allis (unequal knee height) and Trendelenburg (pelvis sags when standing on affected leg) signs

What is the management of congenital hip dislocations?

Treat early with Pavlik harness (maintains flexion and abduction)

Name the most likely pathologic cause of a limp in each of the following clinical scenarios:

Obese, adolescent male with referred pain to the knee

Slipped capital femoral epiphysis (SCFE)—displacement of the femoral head medially and posteriorly to the femoral neck

Painless limp in a 5-year-old (y/o) child caused by avascular necrosis of the femoral head

Legg-Calve-Perthes disease

12 y/o with tibial tuberosity point tenderness

Osgood-Schlatter disease

What type of radiographic evaluation is indicated in suspected SCFE?

AP and frog-leg lateral radiographs of both hips (appears as *ice cream scoop falling off a cone*)

What is the management of SCFE?

Closed reduction (in acute cases); ultimately requires prompt surgical pinning. **Note:** ↑ risk of premature degenerative joint disease

MAKE THE DIAGNOSIS

Newborn infant presents with tachypnea and poor feeding tolerance; physical examination (PE): continuous machine-like murmur

Patent ductus arteriosus (PDA)

1-week-old infant is found to have low-set ears, flat occiput, simian crease, small mouth, and protruding tongue; PE: holosystolic murmur

Trisomy 21 (Down'syndrome)

1-week-old infant presents for routine newborn examination; PE: ⊕ hip click and dislocation of the hip with posterior pressure

Developmental hip dysplasia

2 y/o presents with sudden-onset dyspnea and respiratory distress; PE: ↓ breath sounds on the right side	Foreign body aspiration
13 y/o presents with fever, emesis, and diffuse periumbilical pain that has localized to the right lower quadrant (RLQ); PE: guarding and tenderness in RLQ, ⊕ psoas and obturator signs	Appendicitis
4-month-old (m/o) Black child presents with pallor; PE: splenomegaly and a II/VI systolic ejection murmur; W/U: Hgb electrophoresis shows Hgb S band	Sickle cell disease
2 y/o who attends daycare presents with 2-day h/o of nonbloody, watery diarrhea, and vomiting; PE: ↑ HR and dry mucous membranes	Viral gastroenteritis (most likely rotavirus)
8 y/o presents with painful purpura after jumping on a trampoline; PE: palpable purpura on the legs and buttocks with mild abdominal discomfort	Henoch-Schönlein purpura
5 y/o male presents with h/o hemarthrosis and multiple ecchymoses; W/U: prolonged PTT and low factor VIII	Hemophilia A
Newborn with h/o Trisomy 21 and polyhydramnios in utero presents with bilioius emesis; PE: abdominal distention; Abdominal XR shows "double bubble" sign	Duodenal atresia
8 y/o with h/o Type 1 DM presents with abdominal pain and N/V; PE: Kussmaul respirations and ↑ HR; arterial blood gas (ABG): metabolic acidosis; UA: ketonuria	DKA
7 y/o female presents with breast buds and monthly vaginal bleeding; PE: height and weight >>95th percentile, full pubic and axillary hair; Hand XR shows advanced bone age	Precocious puberty
8 y/o with h/o sickle cell disease presents with severe abdominal pain associated with nausea/vomiting	Vasoocclusive pain crisis

1 y/o presents with irritability plus crampy, intermittent abdominal pain with diarrhea; PE: tubular, "sausage-like mass" and guaiac ⊕ stools	Intussusception
5 y/o presents with recurrent upper respiratory infection (URIs) and steatorrhea; PE: nasal polyps and failure to thrive; Sweat chloride test >60mEq/L	Cystic fibrosis (CF)
14 y/o male presents with gynecomastia; PE: tall male with a small phallus and small testes	Klinefelter's syndrome
4 y/o presents with new-onset weight loss, polyphagia and polyuria; PE: dehydration; W/U: glucose = 400 mg/dL	Type 1 diabetes mellitus (newly diagnosed)
13 y/o obese male presents with a painful limp; Frog-leg XR shows epiphyseal displacement	SCFE
10 y/o with h/o sickle cell disease presents in respiratory distress; W/U: ↓ hematocrit and ↓ O_2 saturation	Acute chest syndrome
2 y/o presents with painless, rectal bleeding; Radionuclide scan reveals ectopic gastric mucosa proximal to the ileocecal valve	Meckel's diverticulum
2 y/o presents with ear pulling; PE: fever, TM is erythematous and bulging without a Light reflex	Acute OM
12 y/o presents with leg pain; PE: localized swelling over distal femur; W/U: ↑ alkaline phosphatase; XR: lytic bone lesion with a "sunburst" appearance	Osteosarcoma
1 m/o infant with no significant medical history presents for routine checkup; PE: III/VI harsh, holosystolic murmur heard best at the left lower sternal border	Ventricular septal defect
1-day-old female presents with ambiguous genitalia on newborn examination; W/U: hyponatremia, hyperkalemia, hypoglycemia, and ↑ 17-hydroxyprogesterone	Congenital adrenal hyperplasia

4 y/o male with a 1 week h/o fever, pallor, headache, and bone tenderness; PE: fever, HSM, and generalized nontender lymphadenopathy; W/U; peripheral blood smear (PBS) reveals absolute lymphocytosis with abundant lymphoblasts	Acute lymphoblastic leukemia
4 y/o presents with barky cough and rhinorrhea; PE: fever, inspiratory stridor; XR: "steeple sign"	Croup
8 y/o with h/o bowel and bladder dysfunction presents for checkup; PE: tuft of hair over lower back, scoliosis	Spina bifida occulta
5 y/o presents with 6-day h/o high fevers; PE: conjunctivitis with limbal sparing, adenitis, "strawberry tongue," and fissured lips; W/U: ↑ platelet, ↓ hematocrit	Kawasaki disease
6 y/o child presents after episodes of "daydreaming" in class which described as "blank-stares"; W/U: EEG reveals three-per-second spike and wave pattern	Absence seizure
3 y/o presents with recurrent UTIs; vesicoureterogram reveals abnormally placed ureteral insertion into the bladder	Vesicoureteral reflux
4 y/o presents with periorbital edema; PE: also reveals swelling at the ankles; W/U: hyperlipidemia and 4+ proteinuria on UA	Minimal change disease
8 y/o sickle cell patient with recent h/o viral prodrome presents with fatigue; PE: ↑ HR, ↑ RR, W/U: reticulocyte count <1%	Aplastic crisis
15 y/o presents with fevers and exudative pharyngitis; PE: generalized lymphadenopathy; W/U: ⊕ heterophile antibody test, PBS reveals atypical lymphocytes	Mononucleosis
1-day-old infant with h/o of prematurity (30 weeks) presents in respiratory distress; PE: retractions, nasal flaring, and cyanosis; CXR: diffuse atelectasis	Respiratory distress syndrome

Newborn infant presents with respiratory distress and episodic bouts of cyanosis; PE: right ventricular heave and loud systolic ejection murmur; CXR: "boot-shaped heart"	Tetralogy of Fallot
8 y/o who lives with 2 ppd smoker presents with persistent nighttime coughing; PE: audible wheezes	Asthma
15 y/o presents for evaluation of primary amenorrhea; PE: widely spaced nipples, webbed neck, and crescendo/decrescendo systolic murmur at the right upper sternal border	Turner's (XO) syndrome
Newborn presents with cyanosis and respiratory distress; PE: right ventricular heave and loud single S_2; CXR: cardiomegaly and an "egg-shaped silhouette"	Transposition of the great vessels
1 m/o first-born male presents with projectile, nonbilious vomiting; PE: mobile, nontender, olive-shaped mass in the epigastric area	Pyloric stenosis
4 y/o with h/o "falling off bike" presents with arm pain; PE: tenderness over forearm, bruises in various stages of healing; XR: spiral and metaphyseal fractures	Child abuse
12 y/o presents with symptomatic, episodic palpitations during exercise; W/U: ECG reveals "delta waves"	Wolff-Parkinson-White syndrome
13 y/o presents with joint pain and fevers; PE reveals a salmon-colored rash and lymphadenopathy; W/U: ↑ WBC and ESR	JRA
3 y/o presents after one generalized seizure lasting for 1 min PE: fever	Simple febrile seizure
2-week-old presents with bilious emesis; Upper GI series: an abnormally placed cecum and ligament of Treitz	Malrotation
6 m/o presents in December with cough, rhinorrhea, and fevers; CXR: diffuse atelectasis; nasopharyngeal aspirate reveals RSV antigen ⊕	Bronchiolitis

15 y/o athlete experiences sudden cardiac death during a basketball game; autopsy reveals a muscular intraventricular septum and significant left ventricular hypertrophy (LVH)

Hypertrophic obstructive cardiomyopathy

8 y/o presents with fever, photophobia, stiff neck, and headache; PE: ⊕ Kernig's and Brudzinski's signs; LP: normal glucose, mononuclear WBCs, and a no organisms on Gram-stain

Viral meningitis

## CHAPTER 7

Emergency Medicine

TRAUMA

List the steps involved in the primary survey of a trauma patient.

"ABCDEFG" (should take <30 s)

Airway—assure clear, unobstructed airway

Breathing—assess chest wall motion

Circulation—check pulses, note hemorrhages

Disability—neurologic assessment

Exposure—remove clothing to unmask injuries

Foley—assess need (CI if blood at urethral meatus)

Gastric tube—assess need for nasogastric (NG) or oral gastric (OG) tube

Name four situations that preclude patients with C-spine collars from being cleared clinically (without radiographic imaging).

1. Intoxication (or any altered level of consciousness)
2. Focal neurologic impairments
3. Midline cervical spine tenderness
4. Distracting injury

What method is useful in the evaluation of blunt abdominal trauma?

Focused assessment with sonography for trauma "FAST" (evaluates pericardium, perhepatic, perisplenic, and pelvis)

TOXICOLOGY

What substance supplements gastric lavage in the process of GI decontamination?

Activated charcoal (plus sorbitol for catharsis)

For each of the following drugs/toxins, describe the clinical picture of overdose and the antidote/treatment:

Ethylene glycol (antifreeze)	Anion gap metabolic acidosis with ↑ Serum$_{osm}$, calcium oxalate crystals in urine **Treatment/therapy (Tx):** Ethanol, fomepizole, dialysis
Mercury	Erethism (insomnia, delirium, ↓ memory) **Tx:** Dimercaprol, succimer
Acetaminophen	Nausea/vomiting (N/V) early, ↑ LFTs, and PT at 24–48 h **Tx:** N-acetylcysteine (within 8–10 h)
Warfarin	Bleeding (↑ PT/INR) **Tx:** Fresh frozen plasma (acutely), vitamin K
Antimuscarinics, anticholinergics	"Dry as a bone, red as a beet, blind as a bat, mad as a hatter" **Tx:** Physostigmine
Digoxin	N/V, dysrhythmias, ↑ K$^+$, color vision changes **Tx:** Manage K$^+$, lidocaine, and antidigoxin Fab
Theophylline	Hematemesis, seizures/coma, dysrhythmias, ↓ BP **Tx:** Activated charcoal, cardiac monitoring
Arsenic	Fatigue, seizures; Mees lines in fingernails (chronic) **Tx:** Dimercaprol, succimer
Methanol	Anion gap metabolic acidosis with ↑ Serum$_{osm}$, blindness, optic disc hyperemia **Tx:** Ethanol, fomepizole, dialysis
Aspirin (salicylates)	Anion gap metabolic acidosis (normal Serum$_{osm}$), respiratory alkalosis, tinnitus, garlic odor **Tx:** Alkalinization, hemodialysis

Cyanide	Lethargy, LOC, dysrhythmias **Tx:** Sodium thiosulfate and amyl nitrite
Tissue plasminogen activator (tPA), streptokinase	Bleeding **Tx:** Aminocaproic acid
Isoniazid (INH)	Peripheral neuropathy, confusion **Tx:** Pyridoxine (vitamin B_6)
Benzodiazepines	Drowsiness, weakness, ataxia **Tx:** Flumazenil (caution in patients on chronic benzos)
Lead	Ataxia, peripheral neuropathy, microcytic anemia (with basophilic stippling), lead lines on gums **Tx:** CaEDTA, penicillamine, dimercaprol
Tricyclic antidepressants	**"Three Cs:"** Cardiac arrhythmias, Convulsions, Coma **Tx:** Sodium bicarbonate (if QRS >100 ms), benzos for seizures, cardiac monitoring
Alkali agents (drain cleaner, dishwasher detergent)	Mucosal burns, dysphagia, drooling **Tx:** Milk/water, then nothing by mouth (NPO)
β-blockers	↓ HR, confusion, possible hypoglycemia or ↑ K^+ **Tx:** Glucagon, Ca^{2+} (stabilize cardiac membranes)
Heparin	Bleeding (↑ [PTT]), thrombocytopenia **Tx:** Protamine sulfate
Opioids	Respiratory and CNS depression, miosis **Tx:** Naloxone (Narcan)
Carbon monoxide (CO)	Headache, confusion, dyspnea, cherry-red skin (later) **Tx:** 100% O_2 or hyperbaric O_2 (if pregnant or CNS dysfunction)
Quinidine	V-tach, torsades de pointes, cinchonism, **Tx:** Mg^{2+} (IV)

Iron	Erosive gastritis, vomiting, lactic acidosis **Tx:** Deferoxamine
Organophosphates (anticholinesterases)	**"SLUDGE"** (**S**alivation, **L**acrimation, **U**rination, **D**efacation, **G**astric **E**mptying) $\oplus$ wheezing, miosis **Tx:** Atropine, pralidoxime
Isopropyl alcohol (rubbing alcohol)	Intoxication, $\downarrow$ respiratory rate (RR), osmolar gap (no acidosis) **Tx:** Cardiovascular CV/respiratory support, dialysis

ENVIRONMENTAL EMERGENCIES

Name the environmental insult associated with each of the following findings:

Osborne (*J*) wave on ECG	Hypothermia
Envenomation may cause local, generalized, or anaphylactic reactions	Hymenoptera (e.g., bee stings)
Type of burn initially causing painless, dry, white, cracked, and insensate skin	Full-thickness third-degree and fourth-degree burns
Loss of thermoregulatory mechanisms, causing CNS dysfunction and dry skin	Heat stroke
Extensive deep-tissue injury under normal skin plus cardiac dysrhythmias	Electrical injury (AC $\rightarrow$ V-fib; DC $\rightarrow$ asystole)
Type of burn causing red, blistered, edematous, and painful	Partial-thickness ($1°$ and $2°$) burns
How is percent of body surface area affected by burns calculated?	Rule of nines: 9% (each leg and head), 18% (each side of torso and each leg), 1% (groin)

Abbreviations

AA	amino acid	AV	atrioventricular
Ab	antibody	AXR	abdominal x-ray
ABG	arterial blood gas	AZT	azidothymidine
ABX	antibiotics	BAL	British anti-Lewisite
ACE	angiotensin converting enzyme	b/d	twice daily
ACEi	ACE inhibitor	BM	basement membrane
ACh	acetylcholine	BP	blood pressure
ACL	anterior cruciate ligament	BPH	benign prostatic hyperplasia
ACTH	adrenocorticotropic hormone	BPPV	benign paroxysmal positional vertigo
AD	autosomal dominant	BR	bilirubin
ADH	antidiuretic hormone	BUN	blood urea nitrogen
ADHD	attention deficit hyperactivity disorder	Bx	biopsy
ADP	adenosine diphosphate	c/s	caesarion section
AFP	alpha-fetoprotein	CA	cancer/carcinoma
Ag	antigen	CAD	coronary artery disease
AIDS	acquired immunodeficiency syndrome	cAMP	cyclic adenosine monophosphate
ALL	acute lymphocytic leukemia	CBC	complete blood count
ALP	alkaline phosphatase	CCK	cholecystokinin
ALS	amyotrophic lateral sclerosis	CEA	carcinoembryonic antigen
ALT	alanine transaminase	CF	cystic fibrosis
AML	acute myelogenous leukemia	CFTR	cystic fibrosis transmembrane regulator
ANA	antinuclear antibody	cGMP	cyclic guanosine monophosphate
ANOVA	analysis of variance		
ANS	autonomic nervous system	CHF	congestive heart failure
AR	autosomal recessive	CI	contraindication
ARB	angiotensin receptor blocker	CIN	cervical intraepithelial neoplasia
ARDS	acute respiratory distress syndrome	CLL	chronic lymphocytic leukemia
		CML	chronic myelogenous leukemia
ASA	aspirin	CMV	cytomegalovirus
ASD	atrial septal defect	CN	cranial nerve
ASO	antistreptolysin O	CNS	central nervous system
AST	aspartate transaminase	CO	cardiac output
ATP	adenosine triphosphate	CoA	coenzyme A
ATPase	adenosine triphosphatase	COPD	chronic obstructive pulmonary disease

COX	cyclooxygenase	EOM	extraocular muscle
CP	cerebral palsy	EPS	extrapyramidal symptoms
CPK	creatine phosphokinase	ER	emergency room
Cr	creatinine	ERCP	endoscopic retrograde
CRF	chronic renal failure		cholangiopancreatography
CRP	c-reactive protein	ESR	erythrocyte sedimentation rate
CSF	cerebrospinal fluid	ESRD	end-stage renal disease
CT	computed tomography	ESV	end-systolic volume
CV	cardiovascular	ETOH	ethanol
CVA	cerebrovascular accident *or*	FAs	fatty acids
	costovertebral angle	FAP	familial adenomatous polyposis
CXR	chest x-ray	FFP	fresh frozen plasma
d	day(s)	FH	family history
D *or* DA	dopamine	FSH	follicle stimulating hormone
d/o	disorder	FN	false negatives
DAG	diacylglycerol	FOBT	fecal occult blood test
DES	diethylstilbestrol	FP	false positives
DHT	dihydrotestosterone	FTA-ABS	fluorescent treponemal
DI	diabetes insipidus		antibody—absorbed
DIC	disseminated intravascular	FUO	fever of unknown origin
	coagulation	Fx	fracture
DIP	distal interphalangeal joint	G6PD	glucose-6-phosphate
DKA	diabetic ketoacidosis		dehydrogenase
DM	diabetes mellitus	GABA	γ-aminobutyric acid
DNA	deoxyribonucleic acid	GBM	glomerular BM
DNI	do not intubate	GCT	germ cell tumor
DNR	do not resuscitate	GERD	gastroesophageal reflux disease
DOE	dyspnea on exertion	GFR	glomerular filtration rate
DRE	digital rectal examination	GGT	γ-glutamyl transpeptidase
ds	double stranded	GH	growth hormone
DSM	Diagnostic and Statistical	GI	gastrointestinal
	Manual	GN	glomerulonephritis
DTP	diphtheria-tetanus-pertussis	GnRH	gonadotropin-releasing
DTR	deep tendon reflex		hormone
DTs	delirium tremens	GTP	guanosine triphosphate
DVT	deep venous thrombosis	GU	genitourinary
dx	diagnosis *or* diagnose	h	hour(s)
dz	disease	HA	headache
E	epinephrine	Hb	hemoglobin
EBV	Epstein-Barr virus	HBV	hepatitis B virus
ECG	electrocardiogram	hCG	human chorionic gonadotropin
ECT	electroconvulsive therapy	HDL	high-density lipoprotein
EDV	end-diastolic volume	HHV	human herpesvirus
EEG	electroencephalogram	HIV	human immunodeficiency virus
EGD	esophagogastroduodenoscopy	HMG-CoA	hydroxymethylglutaryl-CoA
ECG	electrocardiogram	h/o	history of
ELISA	enzyme-linked immunosorbent	HPA	hypothalamic-prturtary axis
	assay	HPV	human papillomavirus
EM	electron microscopy	HR	heart rate

HRT	hormone replacement therapy	MCV	mean corpuscular volume
HSM	hepatosplenomegaly	MEN	multiple endocrine neoplasia
HSV	herpes simplex virus	MHC	major histocompatibility complex
HTLV	human T-cell lymphotrophic virus	MI	myocardial infarction
		MLF	medial longitudinal fasciculus
HUS	hemolytic-uremic syndrome	MMR	measles, mumps, rubella
HTN	hypertension	MOA	mechanism of action
Hx	history	MPTP	1-methyl-4-phenyl-1,2,3,
ICP	intracranial pressure		6-tetrahydropyridine
ICU	intensive care unit	MRI	magnetic resonance imaging
IF	intrinsic factor	MS	multiple sclerosis
Ig	immunoglobulin	MTP	metatarsal-phalangeal
IL	interleukin	MTX	methotrexate
IM	intramuscular	MVA	motor vehicle accident
IND	indication(s)	NE	norepinephrine
INH	isoniazid	NGT	nasogastric tube
INR	International normalized ratio	NOS	not otherwise specified
IOP	intraocular pressure	NPV	negative predictive value
IP_3	inositol triphosphate	NSAID	nonsteroidal anti-inflammatory drug
IPV	inactivated polio vaccine		
IUD	intrauterine device	N/V	nausea/vomiting
IUFD	intra-uterine fetal desease	OA	osteoarthritis
IUGR	intrauterine growth retardation	OCP	oral contraceptive pills
IV	intravenous	OGT	orogastric tube
IVC	inferior vena cava	OPV	oral polio vaccine
IVIG	IV immunoglobulin	PAN	polyarteritis nodosa
JVD	jugular venous distension	P-ANCA	perinuclear pattern of
L	left		antineutrophil cytoplasmic
LAD	left anterior descending		antibodies
LBO	large bowel obstruction	PAS	periodic acid-Schiff (stain)
LCA	left coronary artery	PBS	peripheral blood smear
LDH	lactate dehydrogenase	PCL	posterior cruciate ligament
LDL	low-density lipoprotein	PCP	*Pneumocystis carinii* pneumonia
LES	lower esophageal sphincter		*or* phencyclidine hydrochloride
LFT	liver function test	PCR	polymerase chain reaction
LH	luteinizing hormone	PCWP	pulmonary capillary wedge
LLQ	left lower quadrant		pressure
LLSB	left-lower sternal border	PDA	patent ductus arteriosus
LMN	lower motor neuron	PE	physical examination or
LMP	last menstrual period		pulmonary embolism
LOC	loss of consciousness	PFK	phosphofructokinase
LP	lumbar puncture	PFT	pulmonary function tests
LPS	lipopolysaccharide	PG	prostaglandin
LT	leukotriene	PID	pelvic inflammatory disease
LUSB	left-upper sternal border	PIH	pregnancy-induced hypertension
LUQ	left upper quadrant	PKU	phenylketonuria
LV	left ventricle	PML	progressive mutifocal
MAOI	monoamine oxidase inhibitor		leucoencephalopathy
MCL	medial collateral ligament	PMN	polymorphonuclear

PMR	polymyalgia rheumatica	SGPT	serum glutamic pyruvate transaminase
PNH	paroxysmal nocturnal hemoglobinuria	SLE	systemic lupus erythematosus
PNS	peripheral nervous system	SMX	sulfamethoxazole
PO	by mouth	SOB	shortness of breath
PPD	purified protein derivative	ss	single stranded
PPi	proton pump inhibitor	SSPE	subacute sclerosing panencephalitis
PPRF	parapontine reticular formation	SSRI	selective serotonin reuptake inhibitor
PPV	positive predictive value		
prn	as needed	STD	sexually transmitted disease
PSA	prostate-specific antigen	SV	stroke volume
Pt	patient	SVT	supraventricular tachycardia
PT	prothrombin time	Sx	symptom(s)
PTCA	percutaneous transluminal coronary angioplasty	$t_{1/2}$	half-life
		T3	triiodothyronine
PTH	parathyroid hormone	T4	thyroxine
PTT	partial thromboplastin time	TB	tuberculosis
PUD	peptic ulcer disease	TCA	tricyclic antidepressant
PVD	peripheral vascular disease	TG	triglyceride
Px	prognosis	TIBC	total iron binding capacity
R	right	TM	tympanic membrane
RA	right atrium	TMP	trimethoprim
RAA	renin-angiotensin aldosterone	TN	true negatives
RBC	red blood cell	TNF	tissue necrosis factor
RCA	right coronary artery	TNM	tumor, node, metastasis
RDS	respiratory distress syndrome	TOX	toxicity
REM	rapid eye movement	TP	true positives
RF	rheumatoid factor	tPA	tissue plasminogen activator
RLQ	right lower quadrant	TPR	total peripheral resistance
ROM	range of motion	TRH	thyrotropin-releasing hormone
RPR	rapid plasma reagin	TSH	thyroid-stimulating hormone
RR	respiratory rate	TSS	toxic shock syndrome
RSV	respiratory syncytial virus	TTP	thrombotic thrombocytopenic purpura
RTA	renal tubular acidosis		
RUQ	right upper quadrant	Tx	treatment/therapy
RV	right ventricle	TXA	thromboxane
RVH	right ventricular hypertrophy	UA	urinalysis
s	second(s)	UMN	upper motor neuron
S1(2, 3, 4)	1st heart sound (2nd, 3rd, 4th)	UGI	upper GI
SA	sino-atrial	URI	upper respiratory infection
SAH	subarachnoid hemorrhage	UTI	urinary tract infection
SBO	small bowel obstruction	U/S	ultrasound
SC	subcutaneous or sickle cell	VDRL	venereal disease research laboratory
SD	standard deviation		
SE	side effects	Vfib	ventricular fibrillation
SEM	standard error of the mean	VHL	von Hippel Lindau
SES	socioeconomic status	VLDL	very low-density lipoprotein
SGOT	serum glutamic oxaloacetic transaminase	VMA	vanillylmandelic acid

V/Q	ventilation/perfusion ratio	5-HIAA	5-hydrocyindoleacetic acid
VSD	ventricular septal defect	5-HT	5-hydroxytryptamine
vWF	von Willebrand factor		(serotonin)
VZV	varicella-zoster virus	↑	High *or* increases
WBC	white blood cell	↓	Low *or* decreases
WNL	within normal limits	→	Leads to *or* causes
XL	x-linked	1°/2°/3°	primary/secondary/tertiary
XR	x-ray	~	approximately
y/o	year old	⊕	positive
ZE	Zollinger-Ellison	>>>	much greater than
5-FU	5-fluorouracil	<<<	much less than

Index

Obsessive-compulsive disorder (OCD), 180, 189, 192
Obturator sign, 144
Odds ratio, 119
Olanzapine, 189
Oligohydramnios, 206
Oligomenorrhea, 216
Omphalocele, 240
Open angle glaucoma, 169
Ophthalmic artery, 158
Ophthalmologic disorders, 169
Opioids, 183, 184, 265
Oppositional defiant disorder, 185
Oral advance directive, 118
Oral contraceptives
  advantages/disadvantages, 216
  contraindications, 217
  deep venous thrombosis and, 27
  hepatic adenoma and, 136
  hypertension and, 1
  mechanisms of action, 216
Organophosphate poisoning, 266
Orthopedic injuries, 149–150
Osborne wave, 266
Osgood-Schlatter disease, 256
Osler's nodes, 112
Osmotic diarrhea, 46
Osteitis deformans, 99
Osteoarthritis, 98, 104
Osteogenesis imperfecta, 113
Osteomalacia, 99
Osteomyelitis, 42–43
Osteoporosis, 99
Osteosarcoma, 100, 250, 258
Otitis externa, 36, 45
Otitis media, 244, 258
Ovarian cancer, 224–225, 231
Ovarian cysts, 221
Overflow incontinence, 230
Overwhelming postsplenectomy sepsis (OPSS), 137–138
Ovulation, 226–227
Oxazepam, 191

P
P value, 120
Paget's disease
  bone, 99
  breast, 146
Pancoast tumor, 34
Pancreatic cancer, 135–136, 152
Pancreatic disorders, 77–81, 134–136
Pancreatitis, 134–135, 152
Panhypopituitarism, 71
Panic disorder, 178–179, 190
Pap smear, 222
Papillary carcinoma, thyroid, 73
Papule, 106
Paracentesis, 52
Paranoid personality disorder, 186
Paranoid schizophrenia, 177, 178
Parathyroid disorders, 74–75
Parathyroidectomy, 75
Parkinson's disease, 166, 171
Paronychia, 107
Paroxetine, 187
Paroxysmal nocturnal hemoglobinuria, 84

Partial seizure, 157
Parvovirus B$_{19}$, 113
Patau syndrome, 235
Patch, 106
Patent ductus arteriosus, 241, 256
Pathologic jaundice, 239
Paxil. *See* Fluoxetine
PCP. *See* Phencyclidine hydrochloride
Pediculosis pubis, 107
Pellagra, 113
Pelvic inflammatory disease (PID), 218, 231
Pelvic mass, 221
Pelvic organ prolapse, 229, 233
Pelvic pain, 218, 219
Pemphigus vulgaris, 102, 110
Penicillamine, 102
Penicillin, 15, 43
Penicillin G, 41
Peptic ulcer disease, 127–129
Percutaneous transluminal coronary angioplasty (PTCA), 5, 6
Pericardiocentesis, 13
Pericarditis, 12–13, 17
Perimenopause, 217
Perinatal mortality rate, 195
Peripheral vascular disease, 16–17, 147–148
Pernicious anemia, 84, 85, 92
Perphenazine, 189
Personality disorders, 185–186
Petechiae, 106
Peutz-Jeghers syndrome, 142
Phagocytic immunodeficiency syndromes, 252
Pharyngitis, 36–37
Phencyclidine hydrochloride (PCP), 184
Phenelzine, 188
Phentolamine, 190
Phenytoin, 102
Pheochromocytoma, 1, 76–77, 82
Phobia, 179
Physiologic jaundice, 239
Pick's disease, 165
PID. *See* Pelvic inflammatory disease
Pigment stone, 131
Pilocytic astrocytoma, juvenile, 161
Pindolol, 2
Pioglitazone, 80
Pitocin, 212
Pituitary adenoma, 70, 161
Pituitary gland, 70–71
Pityriasis rosea, 109
Placenta accreta, 204
Placenta previa, 203–204
Placental abruption, 203, 232
Placental separation, 210
Plaque, 106
Pleural effusion, 22, 24–25
Pleurodesis, 25
Plummer-Vinson syndrome, 125
Pneumococcal vaccine
  for adults, 116
  in asplenic patients, 238
  for children, 237
  in chronic obstructive pulmonary disease, 20
Pneumococcus, 44
Pneumoconioses, 23, 24
Pneumocystis carinii, 29
Pneumonia, 28–32, 31, 242